BOOKS BY GEORGE A. SHEEHAN, M.D.

Encyclopedia of Athletic Medicine (1972)
Dr. Sheehan on Running (1975)
Running and Being (1978)
Medical Advice for Runners (1978)
This Running Life (1980)

Dr. Sheehan
ON
Fitness

by George A. Sheehan, M.D.

Illustrations by Monica Sheehan

Previously published in hard cover as *How to Feel Great 24 Hours a Day*

A FIRESIDE BOOK
Published by Simon & Schuster, Inc.
NEW YORK

Previously published in hard cover as
How to Feel Great 24 Hours a Day.

Copyright © 1983 by George A. Sheehan, M.D.
All rights reserved
including the right of reproduction
in whole or in part in any form
First Fireside Edition, 1984
Published by Simon & Schuster, Inc.
Simon & Schuster Building
Rockefeller Center
1230 Avenue of the Americas
New York, New York 10020

FIRESIDE and colophon are registered trademarks
of Simon & Schuster, Inc.

Designed by Karolina Harris

Manufactured in the United States of America

1 3 5 7 9 10 8 6 4 2
3 5 7 9 10 8 6 4 2 Pbk.

Library of Congress Cataloging in Publication Data

Sheehan, George A.
Dr. Sheehan on fitness.

1. Physical Fitness—Philosophy.   I. Title.
II. Title: Doctor Sheehan on fitness.
GV481.S4735   1983   613.7′01   83-381

ISBN: 0-671-45478-1
ISBN: 0-671-53020-8 Pbk.

*To those who will weigh and consider
what is contained herein—
and will test it against their own truth*

Contents

Contents

Introduction

THE MORNING AFTER . . . There's always a morning after, when he wakes up to find he's not a celebrity but a sixty-three-year-old man badly in need of his first dose of caffeine. It's a new day, a new week, and he has to go out and prove himself all over again. He says he welcomes that challenge, but his face says otherwise.

George Sheehan looks tired from a hard weekend on the road. He spoke at a sport-medicine conference on Saturday, raced 10 kilometers on Sunday, then spoke again after the race.

"I'm in a fog," he says. "They gave me a standing ovation after that last talk. Those don't come very often—at least not for me. But I can't remember what I said to deserve it."

Like a runner who has just had a great race, Sheehan's feelings are mixed. He's proud of that performance but wonders, What do I do to top this? Elation blends with depression right after the cheering stops.

The man with one of the best-known faces in running walks unnoticed through a crowded airport. He wears his all-purpose uniform of nondesigner jeans, running shoes, turtleneck shirt, sweater and sleeveless down-filled jacket—all in varying shades of blue. He dresses this way, give or take a layer, whether he's practicing medicine, giving a talk, or writing a column or book.

Sheehan speaks as casually as he dresses. The tone of his talks and writings is informal and relaxed. Runners are attracted to him the way news viewers were attracted to Walter Cronkite: not because his information is that much different from other commentators' but because of how it is delivered. Sheehan, like Cronkite, calms and reassures his audiences. They feel as comfortable with him as they would with a kindly uncle.

But poke through Sheehan's public manner and you find a man who works very hard at making it all look easy. He speaks nearly a hundred times a year but still gets so nervous before going on stage that he can hardly remember his own name. He writes a column each week for his local newspaper in New Jersey (all his magazine and book work begins there), revising as many as four times—"then once more for spontaneity."

This pace leaves him tired early on a Monday morning. The doctor opens a Tab, sits down to start work on this, his sixth book, and the fatigue quickly slips from his face. George Sheehan is at his best when working. He thrives when he's stretching and testing himself, whatever his medium is at the moment.

He says, "That's the reason why at sixty-three I'm not sitting watching the ocean, which I could do—I've paid my dues. Lots of people my age are sitting in Florida now, but I feel I've never achieved what I could. I haven't run as fast as I can, I haven't spoken as well as I can, and I haven't written as well as I can. If you take less than that view, you're finished."

—Joe Henderson
Senior Editor, *Running* Magazine

Prologue
Why Fitness?

EXPERTS DISAGREE ABOUT FITNESS. For every physician who claims it confers longevity and decreases the risk of a heart attack, you can find one who states that no such relationship exists.

This debate seems unending. Acceptable scientific research on the effects of fitness on disease will take years to complete. At present, neither side can prove itself right and the other wrong. It is this impasse that has led fitness proponents to adopt the slogan "Fitness has to do with the quality of life, not the quantity."

Fitness does indeed give us those qualities necessary for leading the good life. We acquire zest and vitality to face the day and its tasks with confidence and enthusiasm. We also produce creative energy, which enables us to be free and spontaneous in problem solving. Fitness opens up the circuits in the amazing storage-and-retrieval system that is our brain. And it gives us another form of energy, the willpower that comes with discipline and the ascetic life.

So the effect of fitness on the quality of life is unquestionable. The fit person develops those qualities that are fundamental to a proper existence. If instructions on how to live were issued to human beings, those qualities would be seen to be most important. Few thinkers presume to tell us *how* to act and respond. But they are unanimous in stating that we *must* act and respond countless times during the waking day.

Fitness gives us the qualities to make responses and to perform acts in accordance with our highest nature.

The case for the quality of life seems unshaken. Fitness makes a person a good animal—an animal at home in the environment, no longer alien to it but filled with a new appreciation of the body and its contribution to the life of the mind and the life of the spirit.

What should also be evident is that the quantity of life is also increased. I do not speak of future quantity, of longevity. I doubt whether we can affect that, except in a negative way. We are born with a longevity quotient similar to our intelligence quotient. We cannot increase that inborn time allotted to us. We can, of course, decrease it—by smoking and drinking and jumping out of windows.

Fitness does not add to life in the future but adds to life *today*. There it has a measurable effect on the quantity of our lives. When we are fit, we can by definition do more work. The day does not end at noon or at five. The day becomes filled with physical, mental and emotional activity. Because I am fit, I am able to do what must be done when I must do it.

Because I am fit, the end of my work is the beginning of my day. Fitness allows for the full use of the body from sunup until bedtime. People who say they cannot find the time to become fit should realize that a fitness program actually produces *more* time.

Running gives me a body that performs better at everything that I must do during the day. Because of my fitness, I can now accept the Olympic ideal—farther, faster, higher—as part of my day. Because I am fit, I am now an athlete.

Accept that, and you can see the absurdity of saying that fitness has nothing to do with quantity of life. The athlete is consumed with the idea of quantity. Everything he does is concerned with time and distance and measurable factors in performance. And so it is with any life-style play activity; the quantity of life increases. The day is filled with activity.

When you are fit, you fill your day. When unfit, you kill it.

Part One
The
HUMAN
MACHINE

Chapter One
On Learning

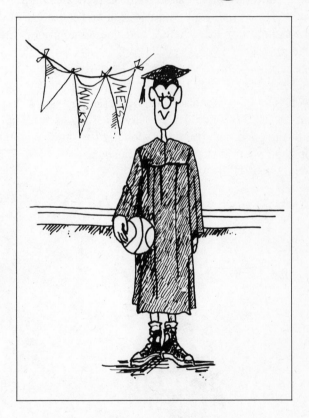

"If you recognize these rules it might not be because they go back to the Greeks and the Romans but because they go back to the Mets and the Knicks and the Rangers."

UNLIKE MOTORCARS and almost every other mechanical device in this technological age, people do not come in new and improved models. Infants born this year will differ little from those born in the fifth century B.C. The rules for the sound body in which to house the sound mind are still the same. In health and fitness there is indeed nothing new under the sun.

Our science is, of course, much more complex. We have discovered more and more of the sophisticated mechanisms that make the body work. Yet all that we know can be reduced to one rule: "Use the benefits or lose them," and one admonition: "Use the benefits correctly."

The general rule has to be applied to a particular body. Each one of us must know what is best for us. By the time we are twenty-one the individualities of our particular bodies should be apparent to us. We should be ready to live our own personal version of the good physical life, following Breslow's seven rules, based on the research of this famous husband-wife team of public health experts at UCLA.

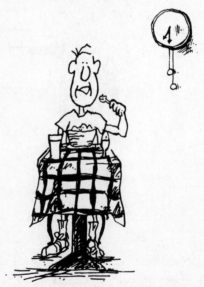

EAT A GOOD BREAKFAST: Culture, experience and tradition have made breakfast our principal meal. Wherever hard work is done, a big breakfast becomes the rule. When I travel the country I see the evidence of that still on the menus. In Arizona, the cowboy's breakfast; in Anaheim, the trucker's breakfast; in Minnesota, the farmer's breakfast.

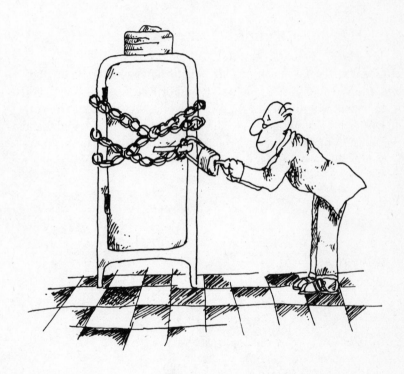

DON'T EAT BETWEEN MEALS: This rule becomes easy to follow after a good breakfast. Otherwise we continue to follow the 90-minute feeding cycle of infancy. For the adult animal such behavior is inappropriate. We are responding to messages that are not there.

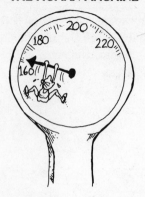

MAINTAIN YOUR WEIGHT: This must, however, be lean body weight. We should not gain in fat, and/or lose muscle. We should weigh what we did in our youth. If we do, we find that the rate of aging is so slow as to go almost unnoticed. Our weight and percentage of body fat are good indicators of how seriously we take our obligation to be fit.

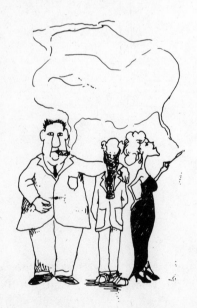

DON'T SMOKE: Tobacco is simply an obvious example of any number of substances hazardous to our health. We should avoid all pollutants to whatever extent is possible. Arthur Morgan, the famous educator and founder of Antioch College, once said he treated his body like a Stradivarius.

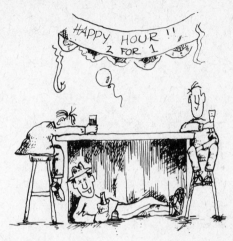

DRINK MODERATELY: Unlike tobacco or other harmful agents, alcohol in small amounts seems to add to life rather than diminish it. High-mileage runners never smoke, but some have as many as three or four drinks a day. The evidence is mounting that two drinks a day may help an individual to live longer than one who drinks more or less. The reasons for this are not clear.

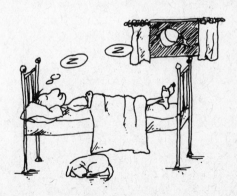

GET A GOOD NIGHT'S SLEEP: Sleep needs are clearly particular to each individual. It is essential to discover one's own sleep requirements. Incorporation of naps, now generally discredited, may bring us additional benefits.

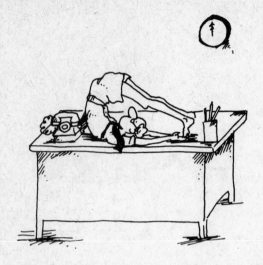

EXERCISE REGULARLY: The fitness formula is a matter of mode, intensity, frequency and duration. We must use large muscle groups as we do in walking, cycling, swimming, jogging, cross-country skiing, rowing or any other similar activities. This exercise should be done at a comfortable pace (that middle ground between hard and easy) for 30 minutes, four times a week.

If you recognize these rules it might not be because they go back to the Romans and Greeks but because they go back to the Mets and the Knicks and the Rangers.

IF AN INDIVIDUAL decides to exercise, or go into training, or become an athlete, just how should he go about it? In other words, what is the fitness formula? What factors go into the equation that provides us with energy and the ability to do work?

Most experts in exercise agree on the specifics. Few take exception to fundamentals of exercise physiology as they are now understood. You can be confident that attention to the following four factors will make you fit.

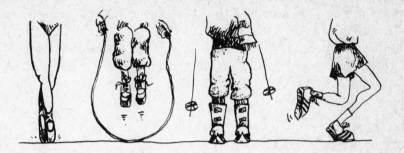

MODE OF EXERCISE: Large muscle mass must be involved in the exercise. The majority of the benefits of exercise occur in the muscles; therefore, the more muscle used during the exercise, the better. Walking, jogging, swimming and cycling are the staple methods. As are, of course, aerobic dancing, cross-country skiing, rowing, backpacking, rope skipping and other activities that might come to mind.

You are looking for stamina, so conventional weight lifting and body building are not recommended. Muscle men do very poorly when they get on a treadmill and go on to exhaustion. Only by turning lifting into an endurance activity, by using very light weights and innumerable repetitions, will you achieve fitness through weight lifting.

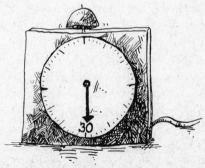

DURATION: The average workout should be at least 30 minutes, with a cumulative total of at least two hours a week. This activity should be continuous, as it is in running and swimming. Otherwise, as in tennis and other racket sports, it is best to have a friend hold a stopwatch on you to see how much of the time you are actually in motion.

This "30 minutes" eliminates any attention to miles or laps. There is no need to count anything except minutes. The training effect has to do with time and—the next variable we must consider:

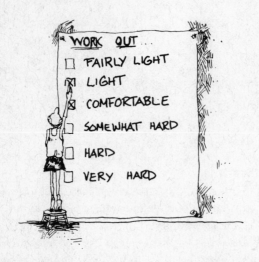

INTENSITY: Most exercisers want to know how fast they should go. At what speed should the activity be performed. The answer is simple. Listen to your body. Go at the effort that the body says is comfortable—somewhere between fairly light and somewhat hard. This factor is based on the Swedish physiologist G. A. Borg's theory of Perceived Exertion, the idea that the body knows what it is doing.

"Most individuals," writes Dr. William Morgan, the sports psychologist, "are capable of rating the perceptual cost of physical work in an accurate, precise and consistent manner." Apparently about 90 percent of us can rate exertion better than any test procedure, because this perception involves processes that are not as yet accessible to our technology.

So when you exercise use Perceived Exertion. Dial your body to comfortable. Put it on automatic pilot, and then forget what you are doing. If this is all too new to you, you could also start by using the "Talk Test": the ability to converse comfortably with a companion and exercise at the same time. This will keep you in the correct aerobic range until you relearn the ability to read your own body.

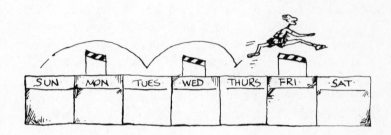

FREQUENCY: The usual recommendation is to exercise every other day. This gives the body a chance to recoup. Glycogen replacement in the muscles will usually take 48 hours. Other neuroendocrine stresses probably take this long to adapt as well. Rest, as Olympic runner Noel Carroll has pointed out, is when the training effect takes place in the body. This is the time when the body adapts to the applied stress.

I prefer going 45 minutes or so instead of 30. My mind seems to open up more with the longer runs. When I stop at 30 minutes I feel I am missing something. So I usually do 45 minutes or an hour, two or three times a week. A friend of mine (a walker) once told me of similar feelings. "The first 30 minutes is for my body," she said. "The second 30 minutes is for my soul."

Running is a low-budget sport. Except for shoes everything you need is already in the house. Once you have bought a good pair of shoes the only other expense should be entry fees. The total outlay for the year should average little more than pennies a day.

It will, but only if you learn to deal with your injuries. Running is an inexpensive pursuit on paper, but not on the roads. Once mileage builds up, most runners develop injuries. And most injuries develop doctor's bills. Costs begin to mount. In the course of treating shin splints or runner's knee a person can run the gamut of health care specialists and incur bills that exceed the monthly rent.

I follow two rules in treating my running injuries. First, I treat myself. I do this even though I could see my colleagues without charge. I have discovered that I know more than they do. Not because I am a physician but because I am an experienced runner and now know things I was not taught in medical school. Given some surgical felt and a pair of scissors, I can shape any number of devices to put in my shoes and help my troubles.

I have also discovered a number of materials and appliances that have been useful in treating my various injuries and overuse syndromes. A little diligent searching in drug stores, running shops and surgical supply houses has uncovered most of the equipment I have used over the years. A partial listing would include the following:

ARCH SUPPORTS: These range from Dr. Scholl's Flexos available in drug stores to the heavier and more expensive ones displayed in shoe stores and surgical supply places. Dr. Scholl's 610's, Spenco and other serviceable ones are generally available.

ORTHOTICS: These differ from arch supports in providing correct placement at all points of the foot strike. They are especially needed when pronation is severe. Mine are made for me by a sports podiatrist. There are however cheaper over-the-counter ones available.

SHOCK ABSORBERS: The first and still the favorite is the Spenco innersole. A new entrant untried by me is sorbothane, a much heavier material.

HEEL LIFTS: I avoid compressible sponge rubber. Mostly I use surgical felt, which tends to bottom out but usually not before it has done its job. For permanent heel lifts inside the shoes, the best are leather, available in shoe repair shops.

AIR STIRRUPS: These new and quite marvelous devices allow a person to run with a sprain or even a stress fracture. They cast the leg, preventing lateral movement but allowing both plantar and dorsiflexion.

KNEE STRAP: Another new and effective device. A simple band that goes just below the kneecap and reduces symptoms in most knee problems. It acts on the same principle as the tennis elbow strap. It reduces the movement of the patellar tendon.

ZONAS TAPE: Made by Johnson and Johnson and not sold in drug stores. It must be obtained at surgical supply houses. It tears easily, molds to the skin and is superb for the treatment and prevention of blisters.

TINCTURE OF BENZOIN: This is sticky stuff that can be sprayed on the skin before you apply the tape.

HEEL COUNTER SUPPORTS: These are plastic bands that can be cemented around the heel of the shoe to give better protection against pronation. They can convert a shoe from being the cause of the injury into becoming the cure.

HOT AND COLD PACKS: To be used on injured area before (hot) and after (cold) running. Just as good, and perhaps better, is the ice-massage Popsicle you can make yourself with a paper cup and a tongue depressor placed in the freezer.

SAND WEIGHTS: These are a luxury but do make strengthening exercises for the shin and quads more convenient and a lot easier. Much less awkward than the paint can, the usual home trainer.

SACROGARD: A small sacroiliac belt for about $10 which maintains the pelvis in proper position. No replacement for a girdle of muscles but will do part of the job until you do the rest.

✓ SURGICAL FELT: With this and a pair of scissors you can become your own podiatrist. You can make almost anything needed to support the foot. These can then be taped to the foot or a Spenco innersole.

The self-treating runner may use all this equipment and fail to make the one change necessary for relief. A change in shoes. I have found that when these measures fail it is usually the shoes that have caused the problem. The heels are worn down, or the heel no longer controls the foot. Getting a shoe with excellent rear foot control can be decisive.

My second rule? If these efforts fail, see the best. I go to someone who has learned how to treat injured runners through treating thousands of injured runners. The books on this have yet to be written. It is worth the travel and the expense to see the expert.

It pays, as they say, in the long run.

Chapter Two
On
Planning

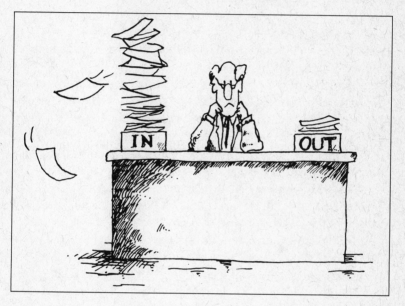

"How many of us put things off, living
for a future when we will have more time?
How many of us live on the allotted
24 hours a day? How many are waiting
for a new day with more time?"

IN 1910, ARNOLD BENNETT wrote a book on "the daily miracle," our supply of time. We wake in the morning, and our day is magically filled with 24 hours. No one can take it from you, and no one receives more or less than you receive. Genius is not rewarded with even an extra hour. Time cannot be bought. And no matter how much you waste it, the next day's supply will not be withheld from you. It is impossible to go into debt for time. Tomorrow is always there.

Out of the 24-hour day we have to spin a complex web of health, pleasure, contentment, respect and the evolution of our immortal souls. So our happiness depends upon how we use our time.

Yet how many of us put things off, living for a future when we will have more time? How many of us live on the allotted 24 hours a day? How many are waiting for a new day with more time?

"We shall never have any more time," Bennett writes. *"We have and we always had all the time there is."*

Let us review rapidly how we spend our day.

"Most of us," said Robert Louis Stevenson, "lead lives that two hours reflection would lead us to disown."

At the least, we are haunted by a suppressed dissatisfaction with our daily life. That is the way it is with me. I am one of that band of innumerable souls who are haunted by the feeling that the years are slipping by—and we have not yet been able to get our lives in working order.

Like so many, I find the day gone and nothing to show for it. Night falls, and I have not added a thing. I go to bed, and nothing has changed in my inner or outer world. I rise, earn the bread and kill time. For that indeed is what I do, as surely as if I took a knife to an animal and let its lifeblood seep out.

Time passes hourly, daily, weekly, monthly, annually, with little or nothing to show for it. The questions hang in the air: "What have you done with your youth? What are you doing with your age?" Things do indeed go slip-sliding along. There is no end to the broken promises, most of them made to ourselves. Starting over is easy: I've done it thousands of times.

Bennett proposes that in one way or another we find 90 minutes a day for our own exclusive use. With this one and a half hours, he promises to help us approach each day with zest. We will rise then, as Marcus Aurelius said, to the work of a human being, rid of the nagging knowledge that we are doing less than our best.

Amiel, the Swiss philosopher, wrote in his journal that "the morning air breathes a new and laughing energy into the veins and marrow. Every dawn is a new contract with existence." The dawn, Amiel said, is a time for projects, for resolution, for the birth of action.

Early to bed, early to rise, is good advice whether you arrive home tired out or not. It is, for one thing, the classic physiology. It is the first choice of our body, the natural way to live. Were we to follow our body rhythms, those circadian cycles, it would be the normal way to spend our allotted, unchanging 24 hours. The gradual buildup in our physiological function and then the gradual decline, the flooding and ebbing of the tides in our body, are matched by our physical and mental activity. The closer we get to following the rhythm of the earth, the closer we get to our own internal rhythms.

Early rising puts us in harmony with those rhythms. It is truly a great beginning. Early rising followed by an early morning workout is an even better one.

THERE ARE THOSE of us who are always about to live. We are waiting until things change, until there is more time, until we are less tired, until we get a promotion, until we settle down—until, until, until. It always seems as if there is some major event that must occur in our lives before we begin living.

Bennett rejects that excuse. He asks for minor adjustments, advises that we start modestly. He gives us simple, monosyllabic advice: Rise an hour earlier, bring your mind to heel, avoid the harsh word. Everything that he suggests requires little more than the will to do it.

The psychologist Abraham Maslow, in describing fully functioning people, said much the same thing: "People who are self-actualizers go about it in these little ways: They listen to their own voice; they are honest, and they work hard."

They find out who they are, said Maslow, not only in terms of their mission in life but in other ways: ". . . in terms of the way their feet hurt when they wear such and such a pair of shoes, and whether or not they like eggplant, or stay up all night if they drink too much beer."

That is what the real self means, declared Maslow. These people find their own biological nature, their congenital nature, which is difficult to change or is irreversible.

We must become expert in ourselves; we must listen to our body, learn its strengths and weaknesses, yet all the while refusing to accept less than what we can do. There are great limits, and we do not know where they are until we get there.

The little ways we reach these great limits begin with knowing our bodies. This perception that things are right or wrong is much more sensitive than people give it credit for. Hans Selye, the expert on stress, once said that the thing that mystified him most was how people know they are sick. What moves a person to come to a doctor's office and announce that something is wrong —often when the most sophisticated medical testing is unable to find anything amiss. Science cannot make a diagnosis; yet the body knows that its homeostasis has been upset.

What we must do is perceive the static-free messages from inner space which tell us there is intelligent life there and it is attempting to communicate with us. For information to come through loud and clear, we must purify the body, must conform in every way to its proper workings. Research is always going on in the hope of helping us in this. But more often than not, the research simply proves what we already know. When we listen to our body, we need no textbook. When we are doing what our body tells us is best, we can be assured we are physiologically correct. There is not a single test that tells us as much as the body and what it perceives to be happening.

Maslow's self-actualizers discovered their own individual ways of fulfilling their potential. As Seurat's tiny dots even-

tually made a masterpiece, so the self-actualizers' minute atten-
tion to daily details made their lives works of art. They became
specialists in the only subject that warrants being a specialist:
the study of the self, the one science that makes you a successful
practitioner in life.

This is not to say that success is assured, Bennett continually
warns us. Always proceed with little steps, he advised. Never
forget you are dealing with human nature. Always remember we
want the easy way out. We want something for nothing. We
blame others when things go wrong. We deny that we have
control over our mind and body. We have become civilized animals and have lost the will to survive and the capability of doing
so.

I once wondered why Maslow, when he places self-actualization as the highest need, put survival as the basic one. Now it is
evident that we must learn to survive—becoming that wild, in-
stinctive animal again, seeing plainly how destructive our life-
style is.

We must live on the alert. Then we can get on with the business of becoming perfect.

Chapter Three
On
Changing

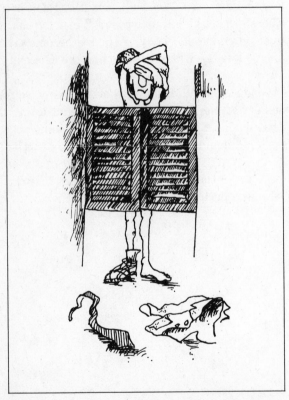

"Once you find something that is playful and addictive and filled with satisfaction, your daily budget takes care of itself. New priorities are set. A new perspective, a new sense of proportion, takes over."

WHEN I WAS PRACTICING MEDICINE and running every day, writing weekly sports columns and racing almost every Sunday, people would ask me how I did it. The 24 hours did not seem long enough to allow for all those activities. How was I able to budget my time so effectively?

It was difficult at first. I found that running could not be simply added to my day. I would not get up early in the morning and do it, and running before bedtime was too much after my long day. Something had to go to afford running and writing full play.

And because both running and writing are play—play of the body and play of the mind—I was able to take my 24 hours and find a place for them. *Once you find something that is playful and addictive and filled with satisfaction, your daily budget takes care of itself.* New priorities are set. A new perspective, a new sense of proportion, takes over. Once I became a runner and then a writer, my expenditures of time were made only when they were compatible with those roles.

Over a period of time, I eliminated a number of activities from my usual day. Most of this surgery was painless. Lunch, I discovered, was unnecessary. Eating a big breakfast left me with no need for midday food. All I missed was the idle chatter at the doctors' table at the hospital, and that noonday chatter became more inconsequential in its absence. Thoreau once said that we should not lunch with people unless we have a new idea to impart. On that basis, my luncheons could be reduced to monthly events.

Movies are no problem. Most are not worth seeing. A year's output in film is reduced to a handful that can stir me to tears or laughter or action. The others are no more than killers of time.

My rules for books are equally simple. I read the classics and prefer authors who are dead or older than I. If you are of another mind, pick up a best-seller list from 10 years ago, and you will get an idea how little of what is current will live on. A classic is a book that appeals from one generation to another. When people urge me to read a new book, I go home and read an old one. There are few good reasons to read novels. Robert Frost said he read no novels because he was too busy living his own life.

The passive role imposed by both the movies and novels puts me off. Like Frost, I want to be part of the action. I do not want to be a spectator. The trade-off for watching and reading is the stimulation of new ideas and the good quotes. For good quotes, books by the great thinkers are the best. Newspapers that contain the truth expressed by the common man come next. Movies are bad, TV the worst.

How many hours can you watch TV without hearing a remark clever and witty and insightful enough to repeat, much less treasure? How many months can you watch a late-night show and not learn one new thing that will change or illuminate your life?

My rules for budgeting my 24 hours are simple. No lunch, no novels, little TV, a rare movie, few magazines, a quick pass through the newspaper. Thus I reduce those hours in which I am a consumer and a spectator and increase the time when I am living my own life.

DO NOT UNDERESTIMATE THE DIFFICULTY of turning over a new leaf. Be aware that even minor changes in our daily routine are resisted by forces as powerful as any commitment we can make.

We believe that change is a matter of willpower. Once we become determined enough, once a truly firm decision has been made, the new life will take place.

It doesn't work that way. It is true that we have to recognize the need for a change, true also that we must make the pledge to do it, true always that such a commitment follows observation and judgment. But *no matter how long and proper the preparation, no matter how strong and enduring the motivation, we cannot add a new activity to our life without taking something else out.*

Should I decide that I want to become fit and I am currently using up my allotted hours a day, then I must take something out of that day to make room for my new thing—in this case fitness.

Why not add it to the end of the day or the beginning? Because removing time from sleep ultimately fails. It does happen, particularly in the beginning of an athletic program, that less sleep is required because of less fatigue. But as activity increases, so does the need for sleep.

Nor is it easy to decide what is to be thrown away. We have to decide between good things, not good and bad. We have a surfeit of riches. Each has value, each is worth doing. But decide we must. Either we choose the status quo and our feeling of missing out, or we break the pattern and change course.

Whatever success you will have will begin with giving up something presently in your life for the new activity. Just how difficult this can be is seen from an analogy with government.

When Jerry Brown was running for governor of California, he campaigned on reduced government spending and elimination of unnecessary jobs. When he became governor, he suddenly discovered how difficult this was to do. Every job, regardless of its importance, had its constituency—people and groups ready to battle anyone who would change the status quo. Eventually Brown saw that the only way to decrease or eliminate a government job was to have a new one created in the private sector.

So too with human potential. You have to learn that everything you do every day has a deep-seated reason. It gratifies a need and offers psychological support. Therefore, begin where the rewards of the new activity can clearly outweigh what is being sacrificed.

"A PRIG" says the *American Heritage Dictionary*, is "a person regarded as overprecise, affectedly arrogant, smug, or narrow-minded." Many fitness addicts become prigs. They pass through that obnoxious stage, attempting to proselytize those mired in physical sin. Prigs become arrogant about their resting pulse, boastful about their weight loss, and insufferable about their weekly mileage or laps of the pool. If their attitude is not holier-than-thou, it most certainly is better-than-you. Their reaction to their nonexercising brethren ranges from contempt to condescension.

One's failures in other areas—creative, mental and spiritual—

the eternal battle with self and a sense of humor should be the best antidotes to this attitude. It will be found that in taking care of oneself one has quite all to do.

Putting arrogance and self-satisfaction aside, there is still the danger of allowing a fitness schedule to run you. It must be respected, not worshipped. Such a daily program is not a religion. Born-again athletes come late to this realization. The sport, first a passion, becomes a duty. The mental exercise, the other part of the schedule, becomes sacrosanct. Nothing is allowed to interfere. No deviation is permitted.

Simply following a schedule risks the danger of looking ahead to your next programmed activity. This is part of the "hurry sickness" and a form of living in the future. One becomes product-centered instead of concentrating on the process.

The beginning athlete, thinker, hero, saint, has to skirt many dangers—almost all of them a matter of attitude. It is entirely within my power—without moving from my desk, without indeed moving a muscle—to cast out priggishness. It may return in a few minutes, but at least I understand how this can be done and what effort it entails.

So too with letting my daily program become an obsession. It may come to rule my life, to make me its slave rather than master. A successful rebellion against this conformity can be made in a rocking chair. Tyranny can be conquered in the mind.

The drive to live in the future may be strong but no stronger than that available concentration of attention we call willpower. Living in the present is our primary aim. Once we make that our focus, we can avoid the trap of thinking ahead—of living in a delusion.

But all these dangers presuppose an initially successful program. They are the dangers of success while the chief danger is the risk of failure at the commencement of a program. Your chance to change your life may well go aglimmering before your plans ever really get underway.

You will never have a chance to be a born-again prig if you don't first become an athlete. Nor will you gain in your mental and creative and spiritual life if the initial phases of such training are a failure.

The rule, then, is to begin modestly. Do not talk about what you are going to do; simply begin. Being born again can mean crawling before you walk and walking before you run.

What exactly is my goal physically? What should I aim for in physical fitness? Like almost everything else in life, it depends on what I am called to be. How will I best express myself through my body? I am looking, in a real sense, for my physical profession—just as I am my creative and mental and spiritual profession. We cannot all be professional athletes—but to a degree each one of us is an athlete; each is capable of becoming fit.

I express myself with and through my body. I am called to be the body I become. My profession is how my body plays, what becomes my body's sport. So my physical education is no less important than any other part of my education. And the physical manifestation of myself deserves, indeed *requires*, equal time with my other functions.

I will be fit because I must. I will find my sport because without it I will be incomplete. If I am fortunate I will find an area where movement of body joins movement of the mind and movement of the spirit—and discover that activity in which the subsequent repose coincides with heightened states of being, and affirmation of myself and all creation.

Chapter Four
On Sleeping

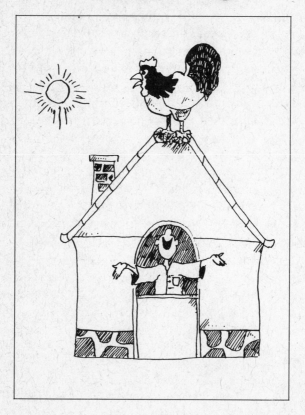

"The human animal was built for early rising.
The human condition is best worked out
when we get up with the dawn."

IN RECENT YEARS I have become an early riser. I have had to. My home is now a large Victorian house on the ocean in Ocean Grove, New Jersey. I sleep in a room on the third floor. It faces the beach and opens out onto a porch with a white railing and a vista of ocean and sky.

The sun rises in that room. All I can see when I am awakened by that enormous light is the new day coming up in the east.

There is no sleeping from then on. The sun and light and sky will not permit it. Their brightness fills my mind as it fills my senses. Not only the flesh but the spirit as well is awakened in those moments that herald another miracle to be.

The sun is a clarion that sends out a message heard in every cell of my body. And it has the same effect on others in our town. Before too long, I see walkers and runners and cyclists out on the boardwalk. In the few minutes it takes for me to don my bathing suit and plunge into the ocean, people have their dogs on the leash and are out for their morning stroll.

Given the proper circumstances, we tend to follow the cycle of the day, of light and dark, as naturally and unconsciously as do the animals. We respond in our efforts and energies as the animals we are. My life in Ocean Grove has proven that.

It is an older community, a town of senior citizens—which may be a factor. With age comes wisdom and a need of economy. Time is getting short; it must be used well. Energy is not as plentiful; it must be used efficiently. Conformity to the rules of nature becomes imperative when you get a bit older.

Some wags call this town "Ocean Grave." No life there, they say. True, we have no bars, no discos, very little noise. The cars give way to pedestrians. But then we are a walking town; we old folks keep moving. Our boardwalk is alive. From dawn to sundown, there is always a parade—singly or in groups, on foot and on bicycles—of people keeping their minds and bodies in motion.

The day that begins early also ends early. On week nights, there are band concerts and sing-alongs. They end a little after nine o'clock, and by 10 P.M. there is very little stirring. Lights start going out all over town.

When we moved to Ocean Grove, our friends thought I had

gone mad. My children took off and got their own apartments. What was the sense of living in an anachronism, a town still living as people did almost 100 years ago? This little hamlet, a square mile wide with all the gingerbread Victorians and the American flags, was a museum piece—not a place to make a life.

But Ocean Grove is more than a historic site. It represents a normal functioning in nature, much the same way the wetlands and the pine barrens do. It and its ways must be preserved. The customs and practices in the Grove are part of our ecology. Rising with the sun, the early morning walk or run or cycle, the pace that allows for meditation—all are necessities to the practice of living. Simple, plain food served three times a day is another part of the daily schedule. I rarely see a smoker. What drinking is done is in moderation.

Dull you might say. I find it otherwise. The days are full. And in the early evening, porches are filled with people in lively conversation. My neighbors, whatever their age, are independent and energetic. They are filled with enthusiasm. They give this little seaside town a feeling of movement I never felt anywhere else. I lived before in a suburb where I was frequently the only person on the roads. Visitors frequently stopped me on my run to get directions, because there were no other signs of life in the town.

But more than anything else, living in Ocean Grove has returned my body-mind to its natural schedule. I am responding to those tides that have ebbed and flowed since my birth. My body is now in unison with those cycles that follow the turning of the earth.

The human machine, the body-mind complex, operates on a program set by the most sophisticated computer ever devised. This human machine is a marvelous integration of innumerable changes occurring progressively during 24 hours. We need not and mostly do not conform to its schedule. But when we do, we are conforming exactly to our nature.

The human animal was built for early rising. The human condition is best worked out when we get up with the dawn.

ONE OF THE JOYS of aging is sleep. As I grow older my sleep has become a delight. I no longer approach my bed with the reluctance of youth and even middle age. I cannot wait to stretch out my limbs, put my body at rest, and enjoy the workings of my mind.

What I have come to treasure is not so much the sleep but the getting to sleep. As they grow older, many people complain about difficulty in falling asleep, only to be then awakened sometime during the night. They now have periods of wakefulness for various reasons. Trips to the bathroom for one. Nagging back for another. I find such interruptions no annoyance at all. They afford me another opportunity to repeat the thinking process that occurred before I went to sleep.

For me this time before sleep has become very special. Next to running, it is my best time for thinking. I have this essay I am writing. I have the information. I have already written pages of words and sentences and paragraphs. I have one problem. I do not know the first word, the first sentence, the first paragraph. I do not yet know the theme, and how to introduce it.

So I lie there letting this consciousness stream past me. I lie there searching for the few sentences that will contain the fullness of the essay when it is completed. Usually, of course, sleep intervenes. I sink down still hunting for that elusive opening. Oblivion comes with my task not yet accomplished.

Then age intervenes. I am awakened, for whatever reason, and once more I can search for the opening that contains everything that will follow. And again I go off to sleep still in this pursuit.

Who would complain about such good fortune? Too much time is spent in sleep anyway. We need, to be sure, the refreshment and energy it supplies. We require sleep to store memories and fill our subconscious. We must have sleep to replenish the zest and enthusiasm that have dwindled away during the previous day.

But must we use up so many hours to accomplish this replenishment? Sleep, it seems, demands much for what it gives. One third of my life spent with unconsciousness. One third of my time on earth in a coma. The only true benefit being that twilight zone before it finally takes over my existence.

If I must sleep eight hours, then these interruptions and repetitions, this twilight zone, are its recompense. These are the times for words and phrases and the absolutely right sentences. These are the times for Eliot's "Raids on the inarticulate." Words always fail but less so in those free-flowing periods between the light of day and the dark of sleep.

So there is nothing that gives me more pleasure than a bad night's sleep. Those hours I spent in bed now have something to show for them in the morning. I may sacrifice some benefits during those waking periods. I may lose out on some of the biochemical and metabolic effects of the various stages of sleep. What I gain is more than worth the loss. I have plundered my memory and subconscious and come back with material I did not know was there.

The absolute quiet for sleep is an effective setting for the creative impulse. It offers a peace and solitude rarely present during the rest of the day. "I have often said," wrote Pascal, "that all the troubles of man come from him not knowing how to sit still." I could extend that to being still before sleep.

When I was younger I either fought sleep or sought it. I never accepted. Age has brought with it that relaxed concentration that makes the best of whatever the circumstances.

Like everything else in life sleep is a very complex maneuver that works best if you don't try hard to do it. As I grow older it becomes easier. As tomorrow becomes less important and the now becomes the focus of my life, sleep and its comings and goings contain the meaning of my day.

NATURE'S WAY IS the right way. So it is with our circadian rhythms. These self-sustained biological clocks tell us unerringly what is best for the human animal.

When I get up with the dawn, eat the right food, exercise at the proper time, and retire soon after dark, I am conforming to these built-in oscillators that control my internal functions. The light/dark, eat/not eat, exercise/rest rhythms synchronize my physiological watches.

The daily cycles will occur in any event, of course. In isolations from environmental fluctuations in light, temperature and humidity, the clocks maintain their spontaneous periodicities. I cooperate with these cycles and lock them into my daily activities to get the most out of my physical and mental capabilities.

I know, however, that my body-mind complex can adapt to alterations in this schedule. Should I get up late in the morning and go to bed late at night, I would in time believe that I am the same person I was before. But it would be settling for less than my best. I would have silenced the protest of the animal within. I would be compromising with life and working against my body.

The major ethical advance of this century, according to Thomas Merton, has been the development of the ecological conscience. Ecology derives from the Greek word for "house." Ecology is a study of the interrelationships within our environment, both internal and external. Basically, it is the matter of keeping our house in order. We have littered and polluted and dirtied our house over the past century; now we are trying to put it in order. The same ecological conscience applies to the house that is our body.

In raising our awareness toward what technology is doing to our environment, we ignore what technology is doing to our inner environment. The indifference and arrogance we have expressed toward our natural resources, we are still expressing by abusing our personal resources—psychological and spiritual.

Former California Governor Jerry Brown speaks of the stewardship we have been given for the earth. We have the same responsibility to care for our bodies and minds—and not merely because that is the ethical and moral thing to do, but because it is the intelligent and rewarding thing to do.

Hans Selye, the world expert on stress, when asked for a philosophy of life, said we should practice a selfish altruism. What we do for the common good should be done for ourselves as well. The more we conform to the workings of the universe and nature, the better we succeed personally and socially.

Circadian rhythms are a fascinating subject. They demonstrate once again the truth of the dictum of Pythagoras that we can learn about the cosmos from inside ourselves. But these tides within the body are too important to be used simply for the delight of the mind. They must be lived. They must be acted out so that each of us gets the most out of the bodies we inhabit.

The study of our body clocks cannot be an esoteric specialty for a group of scientists. It is a vital concern for all of us. It has to do with health and homeostasis, with performance and productivity. Yet we do not look, we do not listen, we do not heed. We ignore the information the clocks give us. We are indeed blind and deaf tenants of our bodies.

The Olympic skier Suzy Chaffee once asked me, "It's 10 P.M. Do you know where your body is?" I didn't. I had never inspected my body to see where it was or where it should be. Only recently, with the sun bursting into my room morning after morning, have I discovered where my body is from minute to minute during the day—and better yet, I have enjoyed it.

Chapter Five
On
Dieting

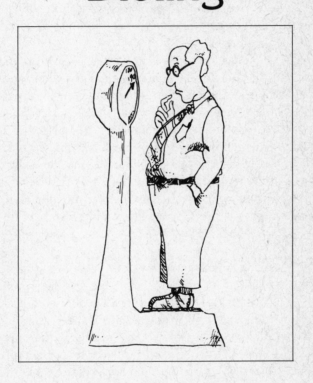

"Millions upon millions of fitness-conscious
Americans are now involved in training and
competition. All of them are concerned
about the relationship of diet and
performance. They are looking for
something that will make a difference. . . ."

THERE IS ALWAYS A NEED for orthodoxy. Whether it be true or false, we look for an accepted dogma, and when we find it, it becomes a fixed point of reference. There must be something unchanging if we are going to occupy ourselves with change. Even the wildest of radicals are aware of this necessity for a bedrock of conservatism. If we are to rebel we want something substantial to rebel against. If we are to start a revolution we require something permanent and unalterable to counterbalance that revolt. If we would have order at the end, we must have order at the beginning.

Which is to say that the rebels and reformers and revolutionaries in the field of nutrition should be delighted that the American Dietetic Association has issued an opinion paper on "Nutrition and Fitness." This professional society numbers 28,000 dieticians among its members; its voice is that of practitioners who daily advise or prepare meals for millions of people. Orthodoxy has finally spoken. Here is a syllabus of dietary truths as these hardliners see them. Deviate from them at your own peril. Which is to say, do your own experimenting, but don't expect us to believe what happens. Not unless you document in it the basic orthodox conservative way every Establishment demands.

Those of us who have been interested spectators of the battles going on over diet and nutrition should find the ADA guidelines of value. We read claims and counterclaims on diet almost daily in the papers and magazines. International experts take opposite positions on almost every issue. Controversy is the appetizer, entree and dessert of every meeting where diet is the topic. The press naturally is having a field day with dispatches from the front lines of these wars about vitamins and trace minerals and cholesterol and any number of things we eat and don't eat.

At such times there is a need to ask, "Where are we?" A need to stop and answer the question, "What exactly do we know?" The ADA has attempted to do just that.

Their statement is divided into two parts. Part I is directed toward the general public. Part II contains recommendations for athletes involved in training or competition.

I find no surprises in the section aimed at the general public. The statement takes a conservative approach that is right down the middle of the fairway. Nothing new here. Just common sense and the wisdom of the human race. It could have been written by Hippocrates. The question it raises is whether or not there will ever be any progress in dietetics. Will nutrition ever add in some new and special way to the good life?

The ADA supports the following recommendations:

1. A nutritionally adequate diet and exercise are major contributing factors to physical fitness and health.

The ADA feels that there is substantial evidence that such a diet should avoid excess intake of calories, fat, cholesterol, sugar, salt and highly refined foods lacking in fiber.

2. Weight loss and weight maintenance should be achieved by a combination of dietary modifications, change in eating behavior, and regular aerobic exercise.

The key is balancing energy intake with energy output. As we get older our energy output diminishes so we have to reduce our energy intake. Exercise allows us to increase our energy output and thereby control or reduce our weight.

3. Skin-fold measurements should be used to determine level of body fatness.

Acceptable levels of body fat range from 7 to 15 percent for men, to 12 to 25 percent for women. However, with well-trained runners body fat is seldom higher than 6 percent in males and 12 percent in females.

The skin-fold method is the most practical test although not the most precise. Even with that deficiency, it is fortunate that skin-fold testing is not routine in the doctor's office. If we had a quick, reliable way to do mass screening for percentage of body fat, America, with all its overeaters, would be in a panic.

4. The generally healthy individual who regularly consumes a diet that supplies the Recommended Dietary Allowances receives all the necessary nutrients for a physical conditioning program.

Here is the point where most opponents of the balanced diet separate from the herd. The precise individual needs for nutrients is the area where most of the fight occurs. Still, it is nice to have that big, shiny target to fire at.

5. Intensity, duration, frequency of exercise should be determined according to the age, physical condition and health status of the individual.

I find this recommendation by dieticians another example of experts making pronouncements outside their competence. Such matters are the province of the exercise physiologist, not the nutritionist. Still it is common practice these days to see professionals style themselves as authorities in another specialty.

This does not mean that what professional nutritionists say is not true. We have to establish their competence for ourselves.

6. The habits of a nutritionally balanced diet and physical fitness should be established during childhood and maintained throughout life.

Everyone agrees to this. The question is how correct food habits, even if universally known and accepted, can be taught. Enriching foods has been the most successful way of getting needed necessary nutrients into the everyday diet. The next best, I suspect, is to get people interested in their own performance as a consequence of eating the right food.

THE SECOND PART of the American Dietetic Association's statement on "Nutrition and Fitness" is directed toward athletes. It comes at an appropriate time. Millions upon millions of fitness-conscious Americans are now involved in training and competition. All of them are concerned about the relationship of diet and performance. They are looking for something that will make a difference, some diet, vitamin, mineral, amino acid or other nutrient that will take them into longer training and better "personal bests." They, especially, are asking the questions "What do we really know?" "How much can I believe about helping my performance?"

The *Journal of the American Medical Association* takes note of these questions in a review of nutrition in the past decade. "It became obvious during the 70s," states the J.A.M.A., "that people in general expect too much of nutrition." While orthodox scientific organizations were striving for "scientific" truths, reports this review, a large segment of the population was supporting the counterculture of nutrition and holistic medicine.

The ADA statement takes the claims of this counterculture into consideration. It admits to some breakthroughs in the nutrition of the athlete but denies others or, at least, denies the fact that they have been proven scientifically. When the ink had dried, the far right in nutrition, those advocating caffeine, baked goods and beer, had won two out of three. The advocates of natural foods, bee pollen, megavitamins and such were still in the antechamber awaiting approval. No substantive evidence, said the association.

The ADA recommendations for athletes in training and competition are as follows:

1. The athlete should meet increased caloric needs by increasing "calorie plus nutrient" foods. The RDA's of thiamine and some other vitamins are increased by increased caloric intake. So an athlete using 6,000 calories a day requires more vitamins. Increase in bread-cereal and the fruit-vegetable group should be emphasized. Enriched bread and enriched cereals should keep anyone out of dietary trouble.

2. The athlete should maintain a hydrated state by consuming fluid before, during and after exercise. Runners can lose as much as 2–4 quarts of sweat (5–9 pounds) an hour. A 3 percent weight loss can impair performance. Symptoms gradually increase with further losses, and a 10 percent drop in weight can lead to heat stroke. Weighing before and after training will give you guidelines. One quart equals 2.2 pounds.

My habit is to drink enough liquid during the two hours before a race so that I have to urinate once or twice. This convinces me I am hydrated. Then I take 20 ounces just before the race starts and 10 ounces every 20 minutes thereafter. Thirst is an inaccurate indicator of water need. A full bladder is the only proof that you have taken enough.

3. The athlete should meet needs for additional electrolytes from foods ordinarily consumed. In other words, salt and potas-

sium requirements can be met simply by diet. There is no need for anything but water and sugar during a race. The ADA recommends foods rich in potassium before an athletic event. As far as salt is concerned, we usually take too much anyway, but a little extra *after* the race may be helpful for leg cramps.

4. The athlete should use electrolyte supplements only on the advice of a physician. This is a corollary of the above. Supplementary electrolytes are not really needed. The recommendation to see a physician is virtually useless since most physicians have no idea of what goes on in a long-distance race or, indeed, of most exercise physiology. However, when sweat losses are going to be great, say four quarts or more, it is probably best to take a half-strength "ade." According to the ADA guidelines, all "ades" except Body Punch contain too much salt, too much sugar, and an incorrect amount of potassium.

5. A high carbohydrate intake prior to competition can be beneficial to some athletes competing in endurance events. This carbohydrate "unloading and reloading" should not be used indiscriminately. It is of no advantage in short-term, high-intensity competition. The ADA frowns on such an intake for adolescents and thinks the full depletion-repletion, unloading-reloading cycle should not be attempted more than two or three times a year. I would agree except that I partially load two to three times a week. After every long race and 10-mile training run I eat Italian-style to put that sugar back in my muscles.

6. There is no definite performance value in products such as wheat germ, wheat germ oil, vitamin E, ascorbic acid, lecithin, honey, gelatin, phosphates, sunflower seeds, bee pollen, kelp or brewer's yeast. Many athletes, of course, think otherwise. Nevertheless, there is no conclusive scientific evidence that any of these substances can help them do better.

7. Beer, wine or more potent alcoholic beverages should not be used as a source of calories, as a muscle relaxant or as an ergogenic (performance) aid. The ADA lists the bad effects of alcohol—among them, that alcohol acts as a diuretic causing water loss and may lessen the capability of the heart to do work —and considers the evidence that there is a better way to get

hydrated and increase sugar store. I have taken beer on occasion before and during a race, but now I find I prefer defizzed, diluted soft drinks.

8. The pre-event meal should be a light one, taken three to four hours prior to competition. The best meal is one that the athlete tolerates well and one he is convinced will help him do well. Some protein, minimal amounts of fat and liberal complex carbohydrates are recommended. This statement yields some ground to the mystical. It tells us that psychology still plays a part in the effect of diet.

The ADA has spoken. This is the known nutritional world. These may be its eventual limits, but I doubt it. Before us lie great discoveries in this field. We are about to find new and creative ways in which diet will help us to cope with stress, increase physical and mental performance, and allow us to explore fully our human potential.

WE WERE 30 MINUTES into Orlando's Tangerine Bowl Half-Marathon, with no water station in sight, when I saw a woman standing on the curb. She was holding a six-pack of beer and a sign that read, "Pit stop for Murphys."

I ran up to her, said, "I'm Murphy," and took one of the beers. Then I rejoined the race, drinking as I ran.

In a pinch, and sometimes by preference, when I need fluid or energy, I will take a beer from a spectator. I know of a few other runners who do this.

The Murphys in Orlando apparently like their beer. So does Dr. Thomas Bassler, the former editor of the American Medical Joggers publication. Bassler usually runs 25 miles on Sunday, taking a beer every few miles. He calls it "Jogging a six-pack." I once ran the Reno marathon with Dr. Jack Scaff, the cardiologist who fathered the distance-running boom in Hawaii. He had arranged for caches of beer along the Reno course.

Still, it would be fair to say I am virtually alone in my willingness to take beer before and during a race. I have gained a certain notoriety by appearing at the start of a marathon with two cans of beer in my hands. If I accept a beer along the way, the other runners instantly know who I am.

I take it as a personal affront, therefore, that the American College of Sports Medicine has issued a position paper on "The Use of Alcohol in Sports." Since I am the rare runner drinking alcohol among the thousands at marathons, the ACSM statement must be for my benefit.

Or could it be that the College wants to stop the revolution before it starts? The strength of a movement derives not from the numbers of its supporters but from the appeal of the cause it espouses. Alcohol has a lot of appeal.

The ASCM gives its position straight and with no chaser: Alcohol won't do you any good, and in the long run it is going to do you harm.

"Some athletes," says Dr. Melvin Williams, who wrote the final draft, "drink alcohol before or during a sports performance because they think it is an efficient form of energy or that it will aid performance. But we know these assumptions are wrong."

There undoubtedly are more efficient sources of energy than alcohol, other replacement drinks that have better physiological effects than beer. I sometimes start a distance race with two cans of Coke and often choose it along the route. The scientists also have been reluctant to confirm the value of sugar taken during long races, but runners know better.

The one advantage of alcohol over sweet drinks is that it requires no digestion and imposes no absorption problems. Some people even worry that it works too well—acting as a diuretic, which further depletes the runner of water. Yet the experiments show otherwise, and the ACSM statement does not even mention this in its negative evidence.

The ACSM tells us that alcohol can affect our physiological tests adversely. Its authors present the following judgments, and I present my reactions.

1. "The acute ingestion of alcohol can exert a deleterious effect on a wide variety of psychomotor skills." (My experiences is that beer during racing has no effect on my running style. It's such a simple psychomotor skill that it escapes deterioration.)

2. "Acute ingestion of alcohol will not substantially influence metabolic or physiological functions essential to performance." (The scientists want to warn me that beer will not improve my time. I never thought it would. I drink beer not for a personal best but for personal survival, not to get better but to get to the finish line.)

3. "Acute alcohol ingestion will not improve and may decrease strength, power, speed and cardiovascular endurance." (There is, however, no definitive evidence that alcohol diminishes performance. My perception is that when I get down too far, the beer brings me up. If I am dehydrated and hypoglycemic, how can beer make me worse?)

4. "Alcohol is the most abused drug in the United States, and a major contributing factor to accidents and their consequences." (The authors of this report now show their real concern: excessive drinking after the athletic event, drinking not for performance but for pleasure. I believe they are overreacting here as well.)

I would point out that most runners are normally two-drinks-a-day individuals. The race is unlikely to change that. A little alcohol goes a long way when you have not eaten in four hours and have just run up to 26.2 miles. I get a nice buzz on after a race with two cans of beer, and I have no urge to drink more.

Beer during the race may not be an altogether satisfactory drink, but it is the ideal fluid replacement. We should never forget that sport also includes that wonderful period following the contest—a time that is filled, as Johann Huizinga observes, "with mirth and relaxation." Try that with an "ade" drink.

IT'S TIME TO CONFRONT THE REAL CAFFEINE PROBLEM. My addiction is caffeine. I cannot begin my day without a cup of coffee, preferably light with Sweet 'n Low. Every 90 minutes from then on I have a diet cola or coffee until I reach day's end and take my two beers and go to bed. The few times I tried to break this habit were halfhearted and unsuccessful. I have never been convinced that coffee was bad for me. It has been an ever-ready antidote for those physical and mental troughs that occur during the day.

Now comes some unsettling news out of Minneapolis. Dr. Arthur Leon and his colleagues at the University of Minnesota School of Public Health have uncovered evidence that caffeine may lessen endurance performance.

Their subjects were 175 apparently healthy middle-aged men. These men first completed a questionnaire on habitual physical activity, smoking, beverage consumption and sleep habits. Then they were given a variety of tests including EKGs, cholesterol, grip strength, and a body mass ponderal index (relation of height to weight). Finally, these characteristics were correlated to the duration of treadmill exercise, the end point being when they developed symptoms of exhaustion and were unable to continue further.

This is the sort of research that interests me. If I am going to change my life it should be for the right reason. We are constantly being harangued by the media about changing our lifestyles. Hardly a day goes by when I don't read or hear that something I eat or drink or breathe or touch is likely to do me in. But these admonitions have to do with longevity, which is no longer of concern to me. My goal is Dr. Leon's goal-performance. If I achieve maximal performance it seems reasonable I will get the maximum out of my life span as well.

Most of the information from this study is not surprising. Treadmill times were higher with habitual heavy leisure activity, especially when it involved sweating and shortness of breath. Such activity was, in fact, the most potent independent variable in predicting exercise duration on the treadmill.

The study group also found a positive correlation of ability with slow resting pulse and low body mass index (weight/height squared). These are indicators I have in common with most serious runners. Running is a leisure-time activity associated with sweat and shortness of breath that leads to a low body mass and a slow resting pulse.

More reassuring information followed. Endurance capacity was apparently not influenced by a number of factors we are constantly warned about. Blood pressure, serum cholesterol, alcohol consumption (12 drinks a week), irregular heartbeat and sleep habits had no predictable consequences.

In these matters we can apparently listen to our body. Within reason we can do what our body wants to do. Eat what we like. Sleep as we please. Take our two drinks a day. All will go well. And those ominous findings we hear about during our annual physical: the blood pressure and the irregular heartbeat and the cholesterol are, it appears, not ominous at all.

What were the factors associated with low treadmill times? What were the life-style practices that most interfered with endurance? First and foremost: cigarette smoking. This predicted poor performance to the same extent that the leisure-time activity predicted the opposite. Then came the same other negative variables: a high resting pulse and a high body mass.

At this point I had a perfect grade. I was doing everything right. Then came the cruncher. Next to cigarette smoking, the most important single predictor of poor achievement on the treadmill was caffeine consumption. An average of 42 caffeine drinks a week had almost the same adverse effect as smoking.

My first reaction was disbelief. Previous reports on caffeine had never contained any threat to my 10-kilometer time. Investigators had written about coffee and a possible association with tumors of the pancreas (now discredited), but they had never even hinted that it might slow me down. Could the old-timers have been wrong who recommended coffee before a race and gave out tea and honey on the course? Was cola something that made me feel good while I was running bad?

My next response was a rush of hope. At sixty-three I am no longer getting better. I can no longer break the six-minute-a-mile barrier in my 5,000- and 10,000-meter runs. If caffeine is good for me, I am the best I will ever be. Suppose, however, it is not me but the caffeine that is holding me back? Rid myself of that habit, and I could have a season of running to rival the good old days. A few caffeineless weeks might make me a winner in this perpetual struggle with the digital clock.

Make mine Sanka, light, with Sweet 'n Low.

THERE ARE THOSE WHO THINK the consequence of dietary affluence is disease. When food becomes plentiful, they say, so does
heart disease and hypertension and diabetes. If the effect of diet
on a nation's health is still a matter for debate, there are still
some results from a country's nutrition that we can agree upon.
This much is certain. A surplus in food has two effects, one good
and one bad.

The bad effect is obesity. Depending on what criterion you
use, the figures for obesity in any advanced country can be
alarming. Studies in Canada, for instance, reported that more
than 60 percent of all Canadians should be considered obese.

Such figures, however, frequently do not allow for the bone
and muscle components of an individual. Weights are given, it is
true, for big frames, medium frames and small frames. These
personal estimations of skeletal size are quite rough and in great
part subjective. What is needed is a quick and relatively accurate
way to estimate percentage of body fat.

My percentage of body fat is around 9. I am 5 feet 10 inches
and weigh 136 pounds. There are others who are 5'10", weigh as
much as 150 pounds and have less body fat than I have. Wres-
tlers and 150-pound football players are clear demonstrations of
this. They are virtually all bone and muscle.

Runners who are thin-boned and lightly muscled like me have
a relatively simple formula for an ideal weight: simply double
your height in inches and the result is your ideal weight in
pounds. I am 70 inches and, therefore, should weigh 140 or less.
And, of course, less is always more for the runner. Now every
pound I lose results in a drop of 0.8 percent in body fat. Should
I lose 10 pounds, therefore, I would be in the neighborhood of 2
percent body fat and ready for a world's record.

For others who are not sure of their bone structure, the ideal
weight can be a difficult figure to arrive at. People frequently
ask me what they should weigh. I have even been asked this on
radio talk shows where the listeners could phone in but where I
couldn't see them. I recall once when a caller, a man, said, "I

weigh 220 pounds and I'm 6 feet tall. What should I weigh?" My answer was in the form of a question. "What did you weigh when you were married?" There was a long silence. Then the man said, "One hundred and forty-five pounds." There was his ideal weight, and there was no way he could get out of it. "Well," I said, "you haven't been putting on muscle since you've been married."

If the what-did-you-weigh-when-you-were-married question doesn't give the game away, there is another one that may. "What did you weigh when you got out of basic?" In this era, however, people tend not to get married or experience basic training, so I ask what they weighed when they were twenty years old. Statistics show that the average twenty-year-old male is about 10 percent body fat, a quite acceptable figure for anyone.

The bad effect of food in quantity is obesity. The beneficial effect is on growth and particularly stature. As the amount and quality of our country's food supply has increased so has the average height of the populace. Records have been kept on the height of students entering Harvard. They have shown a decade by decade increase over the years. The influence of diet, especially dietary protein and enriched foods, on our average height has been quite evident.

The most dramatic example of the impact of diet on stature has been in postwar Japan. Before the war most adult Japanese men and women were of small stature. This is still true of Japanese persons over forty years of age. It is no longer true, however, for Japanese teenagers and young adults. Their average size now is virtually the same as of our own teenagers and young adults.

We knew, of course, that height is in great part hereditary. I know of one basketball coach who always asks his young recruits how tall their parents are. What we did not realize is that the full effect of this genetic factor depends to a great extent on the amount of protein and fat and calories you have as an infant and child and adolescent.

In Japan there has been a profound change in the national diet over the past few decades. Between 1950 and 1975 the average consumption of milk increased 15 times. This means a 1,500 percent increase in milk intake. At the same time there was a 7.5 times (750 percent) increase in consumption of meat and eggs, and a 600 percent increase in fat. Simultaneously, the per capita consumption of rice and potato decreased significantly. And in one generation of affluence they caught up to us in height.

What affluence principally buys is more protein. After that comes the refined carbohydrates, and we adapt to them by enriching them as we have bread and cereal. What we don't adapt to are those carbohydrate calories that lead to obesity.

What parents, physicians, coaches and trainers might learn from these observations is, first, the necessity of protein in quantity for the growing child. The much richer and abundant diet in advanced countries does lead to maximum stature and physical potential. Once that has occurred, then attention can be paid to the bad effects of such diets—specifically, obesity.

The Canadian study showed very little difference in the food intake in those who were considered obese and those that were not. What divided the fat from the lean was activity. Those who were lean were expending calories in movement, either at work or in leisure-time fitness programs.

It was not what we ate when we were twenty that kept us at 10 percent body fat; it was what we were doing with our bodies.

Now you know, what keeps your diet honest is honest sweat.

THE RULES FOR DIET, like the rules for everything else in life, should be kept simple and tailored to the individual. In this respect, we have no better instruction than that inscribed in the ancient Greek shrine at Delphi. The rule: "Nothing in excess." The application: "Know thyself."

Perhaps the greatest excess in the field of diet is the number of books on the subject. Every bookstore is swollen with books offering the last word on diet. Diet books are perennial bestsellers. There is hardly a list of the most sought-after books that does not include one that claims to be the final answer on how to feed your body.

Nevertheless, the truly important aspects of food intake can be summarized on a page or two in our notebooks. Our dietary aims are simple: to maintain optimum weight, to provide energy, and to avoid deficiencies. The rules, too, should be equally simple. Godfrey Fowlere, an Oxford University physician, has summarized them well:

1. The main task is to avoid obesity. This is more the province of exercise. We are not overweight, we are overfat. Only exercise will give us muscle to replace that fat. When you exercise consistently your preoccupation with diet will disappear.

2. Average sugar intake should be halved. Cut down on candy, soft drinks, sugar in tea or coffee.

3. Fat should be reduced to about 30 percent of the diet. Cut down on butter, margarine, cream, fat on meats and fried foods.

4. Increase intake of fiber. Use whole-grain cereals or, in a pinch, Metamucil.

5. Alcohol intake should be kept to two "units" a day (two pints of beer or glasses of wine).

As you can see, dieting need not be complicated. An obsession with calories is not necessary. These basic rules come down to what is now called "the prudent diet." It has a reduced sugar and fat content with some increase in fiber. Salts and alcohol are also reduced but not to limits that would interfere with normal bodily appetites.

In fact, such a diet is a response to normal bodily appetites. It will satisfy the healthy body, which is to say the exercising body. Our eating should be a matter of doing what comes naturally. This occurs only when everything else we do is natural to the body: satisfying the need for motion and activity, enjoying a daily constitutional whether it be a walk or a run.

"Nothing in excess" liberates you from the nonsense of constantly weighing oneself and checking calorie charts; you can throw away those charts of the calorie contents of foods—and the bathroom scale along with them. A school child could follow the nothing-in-excess rule without any additional instructions.

You must, of course, still obey the other Grecian counsel. You should know thyself, know what foods agree or disagree with you. My pre-race drink might cause you to throw up. So be it; choose your own. My allergies are not your allergies. Be aware of this and deal with it. The whites of two eggs contain all the essential amino acids we need for the day, but if they give you headaches or an itch or simply make you feel bad, you must find another way to get those food values. It might be that additives cause problems, but more likely it is some good nutritious food, such as milk or wheat, to which we are allergic. Once you listen to your body, once you can read it like a book, you can forever get rid of those diet books constantly being advertised.

Chapter Six
On Eating

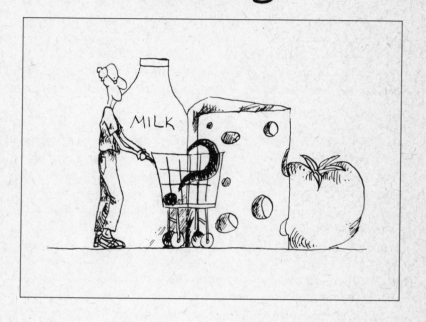

"I look for two special requirements from my diet: first, I must carry the least weight possible; second, I must have the most energy available. The first must be accomplished without losing strength, the second without gaining weight."

EINSTEIN WAS ONCE ASKED if he carried a notebook in which to write down new ideas. He replied that he didn't get many new ideas. And it appears that no one else does, either. There is, as they say, nothing new under the sun. So when faced with a problem, it is best not to wait for inspiration. Chances are, the solution lies not in a new idea but in taking a new look at an old one.

Covert Bailey, author of the book *Fit or Fat*, has done just that with the problem of obesity. He has taken a new look at an old idea—exercise—and has found a solution.

"The ultimate cure for obesity," he states, "is exercise."

Obesity is conquered as we increase our muscle mass and increase the muscle enzymes that burn up the fats and carbohydrates we eat. The way to do this—the *only* way we can do it, Bailey maintains—is to exercise regularly.

Bailey is not strictly concerned with weight. His emphasis is on fitness. His theories are based on Webster's definition of obesity: "excessive bodily fat." People are not overweight; they are overfat. The higher the fat figure, the less lean body mass there is. You can weigh 250 pounds and be virtually all muscle and bone, or weigh 100 pounds and be overfat.

In recent years, efforts have been made to control weight without consideration of percentage of body fat. The significance of this figure in the development of obesity and the rationale of its treatment have gone unnoticed. We have, however, begun to observe that most fat people actually eat less than skinny people. The endurance athlete, a lean and active creature, is often an insatiable eater yet gains no weight.

Our common sense, then, tells us that exercise keeps us slim. The idea that exercise melts fat is part of our inherited wisdom. Still, scientists and nutritionists have never quite believed it. The whole idea seems to go against Newton's law of the conservation of energy.

If it takes 10 miles of running to use up the 1,000 calories in a cheeseburger, milkshake and french fries at McDonald's, the scientists have reasoned, then exercise must be an impractical method of losing weight. The scientific way to lose body fat must be to reduce energy intake, not to increase energy output.

Some people are having second thoughts about this traditiona. view. Dr. Eric Newsholmes of Oxford, an internationally known physiologist, has proposed that the exercised body develops what he calls "futile cycles." It acquires the ability to dissipate calories in the absence of body movement, possibly through the production of heat. When an athlete rests, the wheels are still spinning, still using up energy in these futile cycles. Such cycling, says Newsholmes, may persist for two or three days after exercise—perhaps even longer.

These cycles may contribute to other beneficial effects of exercise, as noted by Swedish medical investigator Per Bjorntrop. Exercise, he says, has a positive effect on obese people even when they are on unrestricted diets. Such people, Bjorntrop reports, undergo "a metabolic rehabilitation." He has documented decreases in hyperinsulemia (excess insulin in the blood), hypertension and high blood fats in obese people who exercise.

What apparently happens is that exercise of the aerobic type causes a hypermetabolic state. When we run or cycle or row or cross-country ski on a daily basis, all our functions are reset at a higher level. We now use the same amount of energy at rest that other people do when they are moving. We are no longer spectators gaining fat; we have become athletes losing it.

Diet alone will not do the job. Dieting reduces muscle as well as fat. It produces haggard people who do not look good or feel good. Covert Bailey is quick to point this out; he will have no truck with dieting. Men of average size, he claims, should ingest no less than 1,500 calories daily; women of average size, no less than 1,200. When an exercise program becomes intense, of course, this intake has to be increased.

Nor is Bailey impressed with pounds lost. When a person tells him that he or she has lost 12 pounds or more on a diet, he asks, "Twelve pounds of what?"

Some of it is fat, of course. But some of it is water, which means nothing. And some of it is muscle, which means the dieter has actually lost ground rather than gained it. This means that gaining weight will be even easier once the diet is stopped.

So what should be monitored if you are overfat and embark on an exercise program? First, do not keep checking your weight.

gain weight (two to three pounds) in the beginning
reased muscle mass. Bailey advises people to
athroom scales. Stop shooting for an ideal weight,
..e says. Shoot for health instead. Become aerobically fit, and the
fat will take care of itself.

The resting pulse, especially on awakening in the morning, is
a good indicator of progressive improvement in fitness. The
change in body fat can be checked by body measurements, particularly at the chest, hip and thigh. These are better signs of
your improving fitness than is your weight.

Fitness tests, such as the Cooper 12-minute test (which measures maximum distance covered by walking and/or jogging for
12 minutes), will tell you that good things are happening to your
muscles and muscle enzymes. When these muscles are tuned up,
says Bailey, you have more stamina, more energy, more drive—
all because of better utilization of food and less conversion of
food into fat.

We may someday discover more complete explanations of
these effects of exercise on obesity, but they will not change
Bailey's basic premise. The choice is fitness or fatness, to exercise or not to exercise.

This is not a new idea. It is much like an old spiritual concept
of which Chesterton said, "It has not been tried and found wanting. It has been found difficult and left untried."

IN 1967, SCANDINAVIAN INVESTIGATORS reported that endurance performance depends upon the amount of sugar stored in
the muscle. When this muscle glycogen is increased by heavy
intakes of carbohydrates, physical-work capacity can improve as
much as 100 percent. When preceded by exhaustive preliminary
exercise, subsequent high-carbohydrate intake can increase the
time at a given workload as much as 300 percent.

This research led to the popularity of the "carbohydrate-load-
ing" diet before races. Now we're learning that runners crave
loads of carbohydrates *all the time*. Such a diet is aimed not at
disease but at performance. It is designed not for longevity but

for longer training; not a lower death rate but lower racing times. It is a diet that is part scientific, part anecdotal and part experimental. My diet has evolved by this process. I read the literature to see what the scientists are saying. Next I find out what other runners do. Then I conduct my own experiments.

I look for two special requirements from my diet: first, I must carry the least weight possible; second, I must have the most energy available. The first must be accomplished without losing strength, the second without gaining weight.

In champion male distance runners body fat is rarely more than 6 percent of the body weight. In champion female runners the figure is usually 12 percent or less. In a study of elite runners in Dallas a few years back, the men were found to average 4.7 percent. That is my goal, and diet must help me reach it. I need enough fat and protein to allow for wear and tear on the body, to maintain body functions and to keep my appetite down. Yet I need enough carbohydrates to replace the 100 calories a mile of glycogen used up in my runs.

What I have come up with is a diet that is balanced in overall fat, protein and carbohydrate intake but not balanced in the way I take them.

Breakfast is almost all fat and protein. They are slowly absorbed and converted into sugar. This is bad when replacing glycogen but good when avoiding low blood sugar. Steak or bacon and eggs give me a slowly rising blood sugar. I am free from any 10 A.M. letdown or the fattening desire to go from one Danish-and-coffee break to another. I may not even have an appetite for lunch.

I run my 10 miles at midday, and following that may have some yogurt and a diet cola. I eat nothing more until supper. That is the meal where the replacement of glycogen must begin; otherwise I will not be ready for my training run the next day. Fat and protein alone can take as long as three or four days to restore muscle glycogen.

Supper, therefore, always includes potatoes or rice or spaghetti, along with fruit and vegetables and bread. Desserts, especially when I am not overweight, become important.

Then before bed comes the "night lunch." I make fair game of anything that can be eaten without being cooked: ice cream, cereal with bananas, pretzels, saltines, a beer or two.

My eating day is then over—unless I am awakened to go to the bathroom. Then I make a side trip for some milk and crackers.

If you run, your diet should maintain your proper weight, give you energy for your training run and help you race your best. It should also be a diet you enjoy. It might even include Twinkies.

NATHAN PRITIKIN is a master magician. He has our eyes glued on his diet. He draws our attention to the dangers of eggs, points out the evils of red meat, diagrams the difficulties our bodies have with sugar, dramatizes the hazards of salt, and inveighs against alcohol and caffeine. He throws a spotlight on the terrible things food can do to you. And all the while he has something up his sleeve—exercise.

Pritikin has always espoused exercise. His plan is called the Pritikin Program for diet and exercise. But both he and his critics have focused on his diet in evaluating the efficiency of his program. And while medical observers debate the merits of his diet and dispute the claims made for it, lean, enthusiastic disciples are emerging from Pritikin centers in increasing numbers. While scientists are saying it cannot happen, it does.

The question is not whether the Pritikin Program works, it is why? The people who come for his help are in most instances symptomatic and on drugs. They have received the maximum benefits of orthodox medical treatment and yet are still living lives that are diminished and restricted.

It is a matter of record that spectacular changes do occur with the Pritikin regimen. In many instances Pritikin patients have no further need for drugs. Almost 80 percent of the hypertensives are controlled without medication. An even higher percentage of adult-onset diabetics no longer require insulin or oral hypoglycemic agents. Heart patients with vascular diseases frequently dispense with all the therapy that has been prescribed for them.

It is also a matter of record that most of this success has been attributed to the diet. Pritikin and his colleagues certainly emphasize it. Our basic problem in America, as they see it, is our standard diet, which contains 40 percent fat and 30 percent simple sugars. One journalist has summarized their attitude: "We have met the enemy, and he is fat."

It would be more accurate, and Pritikin's success proves it, to say that our enemy is fat—not fat in our diet, however important, but fat in our bodies. The problem in America is not food but inertia. And overcoming inertia is what the Pritikin program does well and certainly better than any other medical program in this country. The key to the miracle performed at Pritikin centers is exercise and more exercise.

Physicians who view the Pritikin diet as spartan and austere are usually unaware that the exercise program is even more demanding. In some instances patients are encouraged to walk two miles after each meal along with daily periods of supervised exercise. In his book *Live Longer Now*, Pritikin recommends "roving" (walk/jog) up to 10 miles a day. In the present Pritikin Hospital Plan there is a three-hour exercise program in the morning after breakfast and another three-hour period after dinner at night. His guests are doing more in one day than most fitness programs advise for a week.

This level of exercise has two effects. One, on fitness, the other, on fatness. The fitness equation is 30 minutes at a comfortable pace four times a week. Pritikin's patients have accomplished that Monday morning. Adherence to his schedule results in a superior level of fitness—not mere capacity to do work, but the capacity to do demanding work.

Exercise has metabolic consequences as well as physical endurance. The internal milieu is put to rights. The human machine functions like the Rolls-Royce it is meant to be. Blood pressure, circulation, blood chemistries, the use of sugar and fat and protein are all restored to normal. The limitations of disease are no longer experienced.

Exercise also reduces body fat and, even more important, replaces it with muscle. No diet can do that. Diet alone may reduce fat, but it reduces muscle as well. Dieters lose weight but lose energy along with it. Then, when the weight is regained the percentage of body fat is higher than it was before the dieting began. Even the best diet is secondary to exercise in restoring fitness.

There are good things about the Pritikin Diet: the complex carbohydrates, the high fiber, even the lowering of fat content, although reducing fat by 10 percent would try the faith and zeal of a Trappist monk. A total level of 30 percent would make for a more palatable diet and take care of weight and metabolism as well.

Nathan Pritikin is a pioneer in the nonpharmacological approach to disease. It is unfortunate that the acceptance of his program has been based on his theories on diet rather than on his insistence on high doses of exercise. The reason people come out of his centers looking like athletes is that they have become athletes. They feel better, look better and live better.

WHEN I READ the contradictory advice about diets, I am reminded of Goethe's statement about religion. "All religions," he says, "are true in what they affirm but wrong in what they deny."

There is, you see, no one way to salvation. The dietary experts would have you believe otherwise, of course. Each proposes his way to nutritional redemption, adopting the same attitude as the True Believers in religion. So we see the Pritikin diet and Atkins diet and Stillman diet, each extolling completely different types of foodstuffs.

On the one hand, we have the disciples of Pritikin advocating complex carbohydrates. Then there are the partisans for Dr. Atkins and his high-fat regimen; they form a sect whose rituals include everything the Pritikin congregation sees as sacrilege. Still others follow the creed of Dr. Stillman and accept meat and protein as the approved food. And here and there are various schismatic groups that believe in anything from high fiber to the drinking man's diet. Fads in diets emerge occasionally much like religious cults and are accepted with equal fervor.

In such an atmosphere, I prefer to remain neutral. I am a dietary agnostic. I am not ready to join in any of the holy wars being fought by the followers of the new religions on food intake. I have a continuing doubt about the existence of a perfect diet. I am unwilling, on the available evidence, to commit myself to any single doctrine on nutrition.

I think it best in these matters to be a freethinker. It is best to suspend belief and to admit there are things we do not yet know. There are in the field of nutrition large elements that are traditional and cultural and religious. Anthropologists have shown us that. Several recent books have demonstrated how many of our dietary practices stem from restrictions and regulations set up for us by religious laws.

The way I see it, every one of these diets has something good about it. There is a case for complex carbohydrates. There is also a substantial argument in favor of high-protein intake, even for a high-fat diet. All over the world, we see people flourishing even though they espouse completely different types of diets.

There are the Tarahumara Indians, who rarely see meat or fish and subsist primarily on grain and vegetables. Then we have the Eskimos, who eat virtually no carbohydrates. The Irish have perhaps the highest protein intake in the entire world yet show no ill effects.

So let Pritikin affirm his complex carbohydrates. Let Atkins preach in favor of fat. Let the Stillman faction give sermons on protein. But let them not deny each other. There is room here to pick and choose, room to see the good in each and then use it when appropriate.

I prefer an attitude of skepticism toward this subject. There is more we do not know about nutrition than what we do know. The known facts are a lot fewer than one would suspect. An official in the U.S. Department of Agriculture has stated that we know a good deal more about feeding animals than we do about feeding humans. He said it will take another 20 to 30 years to fill the gaps in our knowledge.

Such statements should appeal for tolerance in a field where bigotry abounds. Yet this inability to hold a reasonable conversation on diet does not absolve us from the need to act. Diet has assumed a new importance. We no longer are interested in mere survival; we are concerned with living life at our full potential. *Our diet is part of our search for the good and better life. We are attempting to live at our physical, mental and spiritual peak. What we eat may well have a decisive function in that attempt.*

We cannot expect everything to be proven before we act. Nevertheless, adherence to a fundamentalist approach that excludes all other possibilities does not seem justified. We must make our own decisions—using the best information, certainly, but ultimately using the final arbiter—our bodies.

I find my body in total agreement with all these zealots in one area. In diet as with everything else, less is more. Too many calories is the capital sin. So before a diet is even decided upon, it is agreed that calories must be restricted and lean body weight must be attained.

Whether overweight predisposes to illness or decreases longevity is still conjectural. But it does sap energy. It lowers initiative. In general, it dims the full light of the day and dulls our sensitivity to all that is exciting and wonderful around us.

Under special circumstances, any one of the popular diets may be effective. There will be times when carbohydrates are necessary, or protein or fat or fiber—or even alcohol. There is *never* a time for overeating. Whatever the diet, whatever the belief, obesity must be avoided.

Here again we see the influence of religion. Fasting or lessening food intake has always been part of the life of the mystic and the saint. There is a saying concerning food that puts it all in perspective: "The stuffed prophet sees no visions."

Nor shall we.

Chapter Seven
On Relaxing

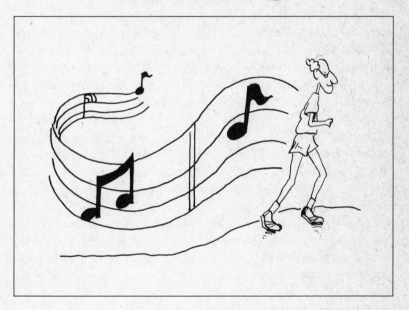

"Exercise has the effect of defusing anger and
rage, fear and anxiety. Like music, it soothes
the savage in us that lies so close to the
surface. It is the ultimate tranquilizer."

"WHENEVER I HAVE A PROBLEM that upsets me every time I think about it," a runner said to me, "I take it out on the roads. Then I am able to come to grips with it without my emotions getting in the way."

I told him I had made the same discovery. In almost two decades of running, I have never been mad at anyone during my daily run. My hour of solitude on the road has never been marred by what William James called the "coarser emotions."

Exercise has the effect of defusing anger and rage, fear and anxiety. Like music, it soothes the savage in us that lies so close to the surface. It is the ultimate tranquilizer. Why is this so? What is it about exercise that blocks these destructive feelings? How does it take us out of a world that is an adversary situation and replace it with one that is one-for-all-and-all-for-one, a world filled with sanity and good humor?

The best explanation, it seems to me, lies in the James-Lange theory of emotions. This is one of psychology's most unlikely hypotheses and one usually given little credence. Yet as with most ideas espoused by James, time gives us more and more evidence that he was right.

According to James, I do not first get angry and then exhibit that anger in my body. The actual process is the reverse. My *body* gets angry, and then I become angry. My body perceives the object or idea that causes anger, reacts with the usual physiological phenomena—rapid pulse, flushing of the face, etc.—and only then do I feel the emotion of anger.

When I first read this explanation, I found it incredible. The truth, as I saw it, was obvious: I saw or remembered or dreamed up an object or idea that frightened me or angered me, causing me to feel guilty or to know hate—and then my body reacted to that feeling. The James-Lange theory was, in a word, absurd.

Now I think otherwise. James seems to be correct. If my body does not react to the object or idea, I now realize that I don't feel these emotions. It is not until the physiological effects occur that the emotion becomes apparent. If the usual signs and symptoms of rage are blocked, then I will not feel rage in my mind.

Such blocking can occur in two ways: first, by flooding the various systems of the body with activity so that there is no reserve to produce the reaction identified with the emotion; second, by substituting some positive emotion in its place. (Act happy, look happy, speak happily, said James, and you will be happy. Act like an enthusiast, and you will become an enthusiast.)

When I run, both of these events take place. Running completely occupies my body. It fills every cell. I am all movement, effort, sweat. I become the running as the dancer becomes the dance. The entire functioning of my body is focused on this one action. There is no room for the coarser emotions. Only the higher and more subtle feelings are now able to enter my consciousness.

And indeed they do. Now I can imagine myself a hero and have my body feel heroic; think of myself as a success and find failure unimaginable; know that part of me is good and whole and true, and feel faith flooding through me. My body takes me through the friendly vistas of my river road to even friendlier vistas of my soul. My mind can now think what it likes. It runs ahead of me, investigating things along the way. It is no longer impeded or affected by the negative emotions my body usually creates.

My body usually creates the typical physiological patterns that I know as anger or fear, guilt or rage. And for me, running is the best way to prevent these particular patterns from developing. When I run, I am absolved from those feelings that destroy rather than create, that lead to darkness rather than light. I am cleansed of the passions that arise when I see the world as Them or Us, or rail against Fate, or attempt to change things over which I have no control.

Is running necessary for this? Of course not. The Stoics knew this centuries ago. There is no better guide to tranquility than Marcus Aurelius, no better antidote to anxiety than reading Epictetus. But for those of us made of lesser stuff, the pragmatist James has shown an easier way.

We have discovered an alternative path to peace and serenity.

We are coping with life—and quite well, thank you—on the move.

THE MOST DANGEROUS THING a man possesses is a logical mind. A logical mind is practical and pragmatic. It knows the price of everything and the value of nothing. It reacts appropriately to danger and inappropriately to love. It accepts work but not play, understands science but not religion. The logical mind ends where a sense of humor starts.

Almost equally dangerous are our appetites and emotions. Unchecked appetites change us from free men to slaves. The negative emotions of hate and envy and despair can kill the good life as surely as a bullet.

What we need is something to synthesize these forces—something to bring harmony to these opposites, create unity out of this diversity, fuse the body, mind and spirit into the unique person each of us is.

Surprisingly, philosophers have suggested that this is best accomplished in sports. "Man at his utmost," "self-completion (through excellence)" and "self-actualization through self-extension" are a few of the descriptions they give of the effect of sports on the athlete.

The surfer is not merely seeking the perfect wave, the skier the perfect slope, the runner the perfect race. Each is seeking his own perfection, seeking to purge the negative emotions, seeking to quell the animal appetites, seeking to keep the brain at work on things the brain should do, but most of all seeking a total acceptance of himself and his universe, a loving of himself and his fellows and his Creator. For the athlete, sport is not a religion; it is a religious act that brings together work and play, love and religion.

I would be less certain of this if I had not read William Gibson's *A Season in Heaven*, an account of his experience studying Transcendental Meditation in Spain under Maharishi Mahesh Yogi. Gibson went because TM had transformed his son who had been drowning in "eddies of self-hatred" into a smiling, loving person.

Scientists tell us that TM is a physiological method of obtaining relaxation and a hypometabolic state. Dr. Herbert Benson of Harvard University has reported a lowering of blood pressure, a decrease in oxygen intake, and a slowing of the pulse while deep in TM. Many other advantageous metabolic changes are also known to occur. ("I had a letting-go inside," writes Gibson, "which was the first waking rest I'd had from myself in 50 years.")

The key to this is the mantra. This is a simple Vedic sound without meaning (Benson claims any word may do). What it does is throw the reasoning brain off the scent while you descend into the absolute—moving away from the stresses that surround you, the disharmony, the diversity, the opposites, all the evidence you have of your mortality. The mantra allows you to get out of that bind into unity.

This unity is the promise of TM: a body free from stress and a mind open to boundless energy, intelligence, creativity, skill in action and better behavior toward others. This result comes gradually. Recruits to this method initially feel an increase in energy, both mental and physical. They make complete turn-abouts as to drugs and alcohol and tobacco. There is even some talk about celibacy. Only later comes the religion that sees God as It.

For Gibson, the religion that opened up to him was his own. A nonbelieving Catholic since the age of fourteen, he returned home as a daily Mass-goer. He was able, he said, to convince his logical mind to leave his nonrational religion alone. He had found in TM a solution to his own conflicts, and also an antidote to the counsel of our best minds—"despair, impotence and self-loathing."

I have also gone the TM route—brought the flowers and the fruit and the $75 required to attend a series of four lectures. I agree with much of what Gibson writes, and I am interested in his spiritual odyssey. But I'm inclined to think, at least for me, that running offers more.

What sport does additionally is to bring the body and mind on this trip into what Maharishi calls "cosmic consciousness," the level where we deal in absolutes only, and because running does that, it takes me totally body-mind-soul into this new experience. I am man fully functioning, and there is no one on God's earth I would trade places with at that moment.

ONE OF THE MORE EFFECTIVE ways of relieving stress is the relaxation response. This is an altered state of consciousness in which the mind and the body are deeply relaxed. At the same time, your awareness of the world and its worries diminishes and you are temporarily at peace. The methods used to attain this state are primarily those of Transcendental Meditation and the technique described by Dr. Benson in his book *The Relaxation Response.*

From personal experience, I can tell you they work. The TM and Benson procedures are simple and, except for the mantra, identical. It is suggested you sit in a comfortable chair, relax your muscles, close your eyes, breathe deeply and slowly with your belly and then repeat your mantra or the word "one." This is done in tempo with your heart beat (if as slow as mine) or with your breathing. Distracting thoughts are not fought; they succumb to the recitation of the word.

To many, these measures seem quite superficial. They depart from the traditional psychological approach of changing physiological responses by unmasking the psychological factors and feelings that produce them. Stress, say these experts, must first be understood, then dealt with.

Relaxation responses, of course, do the opposite. They treat the effect, not the cause; the result, not the reason. What they seek is oblivion, a mind cleansed of thought, muscles relaxed to jelly. This type of meditation is not active or passive; it is negative. It is the way of detachment, of elimination, of emptiness.

What happens, then, is a reaction that prescinds from the cause of our hurry and worry, that cares not why or how we become tense or anxious. There is no need for psychoanalysis or psychotherapy, no need for insight and acceptance, no need to ask the Great Questions or to debate the answers, no need to study our unconscious or subconscious or even our conscious. Just follow the simple instructions and drift away.

These procedures return me to my resting state. When I use them I am in effect hunkering down, turning my tail to the wind and riding out the storm. These techniques give me a respite, a timeout, a period when I can get my breath, regain my composure, remember my game plan.

That last, I suppose, is most important. One basketball coach told me that about timeouts. "There is not much you can do," he said, "except remind them of what they do best."

When I come back from a relaxation timeout, I am reminded of what I do best. I have lost, for the most part, the tension, the feeling of straining, of being in over my head. I have regained, if only temporarily, the rhythm of my game.

That rhythm is different for each one of us. It is, however, always similar in principle. I am, as you are, like a reciprocating motor. Deep in my chest, I feel the pulsation of my heart, alternately filling and emptying. And this same systole and diastole occur in all my other activities.

There is work and play, effort and rest, times when I store energy and other times when I discharge it. The good life is a product of this balance, this alternation that enables me to accept and make the most out of the inevitable tensions and stresses I meet.

It is interesting that stress expert Hans Selye sees no need for these relaxation techniques. We would be better occupied, he states, in taking a different attitude toward the events in our life. Attitude determines whether we perceive an experience as pleasant or unpleasant. It is in adopting the right attitude, he says, that we can convert a negative stress into a positive one.

His criticism is true to an extent. The effect of a period of relaxation is brief. When I come back, nothing has been radically changed—any more than it would be if I had taken a nap. I might have been given time to remember my game plan, but I haven't discovered anything new about myself or the game.

So Selye is right. There may be a place for sitting still and making my mind a blank. But what I need more is some positive method of relaxation—one that is associated with play and movement, with creation and contemplation. So for me the supreme relaxation technique is, again, running.

Selye himself swims or bikes in the morning, then swims and lifts weights at night. These are periods of time where he is, it seems to me, employing his own relaxation techniques, which are quite similar to mine.

What we should remember is that, in dealing with stress, good intentions are not enough. In the final analysis, we need the tools, we need the skill, we need the techniques. *We have come to a time when a person who cannot play is illiterate, a person who cannot relax is a barbarian, and a person who cannot meditate has not yet learned to live.*

Chapter Eight
On Adapting

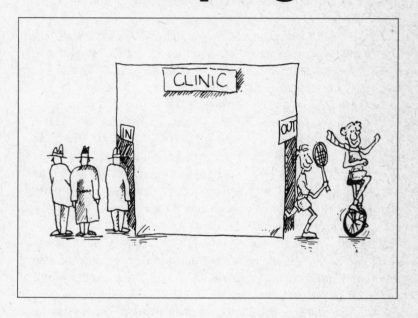

"Stress makes us fit, ready of mind, people of virtue and courage. Stress is what makes us complete. Through it we advance, grow, stay alive—but not without danger. Stress is a struggle that can also destroy."

STRESS IS THE STUFF that shapes me, the force that forces me to do my best, the stimulus that makes me the person I am.

But as society changes, so does stress. We are faced now with less and less physical stress, more and more mental and psychological stress. That is our way of doing things. Man is a technician. He expends effort to decrease effort. He strives to remove the need to work and thereby concentrates on living well. The mission of technology consists in releasing man for the task of being himself.

The result is increasing security and leisure, protection from the elements, a decrease in physical work. A great deal of physical stress has been eliminated from our day-to-day living—particularly the stresses that led to the strength of the body, the maintenance of vigor and the development of endurance.

Physical stress is no longer obligatory. Technology has liberated us from these boons to our physiology. Now we have indoor plumbing and central heating, air conditioning and hot showers. We have transportation that virtually removes the need to walk. Time and space have been conquered. We have all sorts of labor-saving devices. We have even reached the ultimate; we have put men in orbit and removed the final stress—gravity.

Physical stress therefore must be sought. It must be self-administered. We have come to a point in our physical existence much like the spiritual crisis described by Pelagius: "If we wish not to go backwards, we must run." Unless we become athletes, we can never become the self that is our project on this earth.

For each of us, this athlete inside is different, and the stress needed to become an athlete is necessarily different. Mine is the stress needed to become a long-distance runner. I administer it in measured doses of time and frequency and intensity. I run this far, this fast, this often. And then I rest at a certain plateau of performance, readying myself for another assault on the summit.

The principle for everyone is the same: the application of stress, which is the alarm period; then the period of adaptation, of mastery, followed by rest and recuperation. There is thus a general formula for fitness, and yet there is no absolute formula for fitness. The body alone knows, and every body is different.

Training is not a cookbook system. Guidelines work only up to a point. I must listen to my body, know my body's wisdom, learn to reach what is going on inside.

Technique is another matter. There I must go with the best, learn how to minimize stress. So I run with the least effort. I shorten and shorten my stride until it is as if I am riding a bicycle in low gear.

So too I must learn the best methods of rest and recuperation —sleep and naps, of course, but also relaxation techniques and biofeedback. All help to restore and revitalize. All set me up for another day, another try at my peak.

There are always missteps, to be sure. That climb is never uninterrupted. Sometimes the stress is too much, the rest period too short. I break down with a cold or am possessed with exhaustion. Then nothing pleases me. The run is a bore, the race a disaster.

But this only shows that I am responsible, not only for defeat but for victory as well. I can no longer blame chance or fate or technology for the bad things that happen, but I can take credit if things go well.

STRESS HAS BEEN DEFINED as any condition or situation that imposes on a person demands for adjustment. It is therefore a fact of life—omnipresent, inevitable. Stress is a constant presence in our day. Whether it be physical or mental or emotional, it is unavoidable. And should we take to our beds and pull the covers over our heads, we simply substitute other stresses: the stress of inactivity on the body, the stress of guilt on the psyche, the stress of isolation on the mind.

Stress therefore must be accepted, must be seen for the good it does, and then managed so the bad consequences are minimized. It must be welcomed, because with it we would be less than our best. In accepting stress, we know the truth of Nietzsche's words, "What does not destroy me makes me strong."

Stress makes us fit, ready of mind, people of virtue and courage. Stress is what makes us complete. Through it we advance, grow, stay alive—but not without danger. Stress is a struggle that can also destroy. It can weaken me physically, make me ill, cause a nervous breakdown, force me to lose my faith in myself and in creation.

But there is no alternative. Were I not to engage in this continuous encounter, I would give up the possibility of being stretched to my limit. I would give up all chance I have of realizing, as Theodore Rozak put it, my original splendor—the potential I had at birth.

The business of life, then, is stress. By using instinct and intelligence, discipline and humor, a sense of play, a feeling of self-esteem, I must first identify stress and then learn how to handle it.

The principles of stress and its effects are quite simple. There is the first stage of shock or alarm in which the whole force of physical and mental and psychological resources is brought to bear on the situation. Then, in the second stage, there is the gradual return to equilibrium, the restoration of the internal milieu. The whole organism, the person I am, then comes to a balance a notch higher than when the stress was imposed. At times, of course, the opposite happens. The stress is too great, the time allowed for recuperation is too short, and exhaustion or breakdown occurs.

Stress comes in large, small or medium sizes. It can be physical, emotional, mental or spiritual, or combinations of any or all of these. The crisis that confronts us may be running a marathon or passing an examination, a domestic quarrel or a deadline on an assignment, as major as the acceptance of death or as minor as a faulty carburetor.

Each of us perceives and reacts differently to these stresses. This is as it should be. I am a unique individual. My body and mind and soul were made for me and no other. My reaction is in my own style, as personal as my fingerprints. To find it, I must be an experiment-of-one. No facts should be sacred, no other's experience accepted. My task is to know myself, to learn whether I am primarily made for flight or fight, to understand what stresses I handle best.

Let it be said, however, that there are no bad stresses, just as there are no bad experiences. Everything is part of the great experiment, part of the learning process. Stress is a necessity for the good life—that is the first great lesson to learn. The second and no less important is that all of us have our own special way of dealing with it.

I am my own consultant; my own subject. I do not look for advice; nor should you. I subscribe to Emerson's thought on this matter.

"Cannot we let people be themselves and enjoy life in their way?" he asked. "You are trying to make that man another you. One's enough."

One is indeed enough. *I am satisfied to make my own lonely struggle. So in my running and my day-to-day living, I seek stress—but my own stress, the stress that my body welcomes, that my mind enjoys and that makes my soul happy.*

SUPPOSE I ACCEPT the belief that physical fitness is essential to the good life, that training and conditioning are necessary to my day-to-day living. And suppose I do train, become a good animal, an athlete, a runner, a swimmer, a cyclist. What then?

What I mean is, where does all of this fit into the scheme of things? Will this physical health translate into mental health? Will this physical fitness contribute to psychological fitness? Will this ability to deal with physical stress do something to help me in my struggle with psychological stress?

I know from my athletic friends that it can. One friend credits running for his coping with the death of his wife. Others have become recovered alcoholics. Still others have survived long periods of anxiety and depression. And there are legions of men and women who have experienced other affirmative psychological effects from their sports.

There is also a reinforcing reverse evidence. Athletes who are injured and have to give up their sport frequently go through a period of depression that is relieved only by the resumption of activity. Until they can move freely again, they are unable to withstand even the most minor misfortune. Indeed, daily living becomes too much for them.

Why all this should be so is a mystery to me. The problem of the body-soul relationship has stumped minds infinitely more capable than mine. There is general agreement that a relationship, either direct or in parallel, exists—and that it would be best to consider the body and the soul as different functions of the same thing. Whatever happens to one effects the other.

"We often hear," said the late Paul Dudley White, "of the effect of the mind on the body. We should not forget the effect of the body on the mind."

I can attest to that effect, especially the immediate one. When I have had it up to here, when my levels of frustration have reached a critical point, when I know I will assault—at least verbally—the next person I meet, when I am in a situation where the usual advice is to count to 10, I run to 10—miles, that is.

I take off and run until that heat dissipates, and when I get back, I have usually forgotten what upset me. I am pleasantly fatigued. I have what the psychiatrists call a global feeling of well-being.

This response is a complicated interaction of physiological and psychological effects, each relating to the other. There are two ways, you see, to handle stress. One is modifying the physiological response to that stress. The other is improving psychological health.

We determine our own stress. What is stressful to me might be of no consequence to someone else. Our reactions are equally individual. We are equipped with instincts that impel us to fight or take flight—or in some instances to negotiate.

My impulse, which is to flee, would have been in more primitive times, a lifesaving impulse in a life-threatening situation. Now my situation can hardly be called life-and-death. Aggravating, perhaps; frustrating, maybe; depressing, certainly—but not something associated with bodily harm. Yet the body is being mobilized to bend steel, lift cars or leap a wall at a single bound.

Before my run, the body is preparing me for a lifesaving maneuver that has to be performed maximally. To do so, it secretes hormones and, among other things, raises the pulse and blood pressure and blood sugar. It does this through a variety of marvelous physiological actions. But it also puts me in a state that has no legitimate outlet.

I give it that outlet by running. I use these energies in a healthy, happy way. Through my running, I am able to work off this excessive, inappropriate reaction. I am able to dampen those primitive responses of my autonomic nervous system. I regain control of my body in much the same way that a cowboy subdues a bucking bronco: I ride it until it tires out.

Chapter Nine
On
Craving

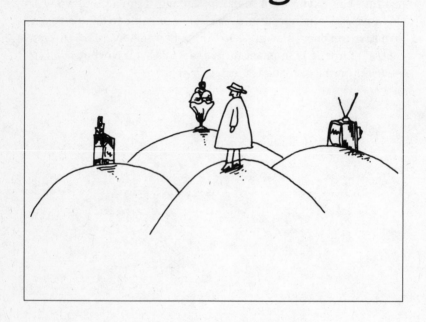

"If you are going to take something enjoyable out of your life, you must put something of comparable enjoyment into it. We may think there is willpower involved, but more likely the change is due to want power. Wanting the new addiction more than the old one. Wanting the new me in preference to the old person I am now."

WHY SHOULD WE NONSMOKERS care about the smoker's problem? Why should we be concerned about what happens to these people who are dependent on nicotine? The answer is self-interest. We do wish our neighbor well, but we wish ourselves well even more. We are all dependent on something. We are addicted in some way. If not to cigarettes then to something else. What works for cigarettes and nicotine may well work for whatever we are trying to get rid of in our lives.

So whether our addiction is food or sex or TV; whether we have a burning need for just one more drink or an extra hour of sleep in the morning; whether we cannot control a controlled substance or legitimize an illegitimate relationship, the principle is the same. What helps people rid themselves of their addiction can help us handle ours.

Freud saw the answer in a substitute or surrogate activity. We need to replace these satisfying pursuits with something just as satisfying. If you are going to take something enjoyable out of your life you must put something of comparable enjoyment into it. We may think there is willpower involved, but more likely the change is due to want power. Wanting the new addiction more than the old one. Wanting the new me in preference to the old person I am now.

One such substitute is running. Peter Wood in his studies at Stanford discovered that runners who put in 40 miles a week on the roads did not smoke. Many of them had been two- or three-pack-a-day smokers prior to taking up running. In almost all instances they began running and then gradually gave up the cigarettes. Another study at the University of Alabama reported that only 3 percent of the joggers and runners interviewed were still smoking. In addition, the cigarette consumption was usually limited to 15 cigarettes a day.

Most of the runners I meet are ex-addicts. The addiction might have been drugs or alcohol or simply a sedentary way of life. Running turned their lives around. In every lecture I give to runners I know there is a story for each person in the audience. Each one has taken charge of their novel in the making. Each one has a tale to tell about what they were like before they began running and how they have changed for the better—physically, mentally and spiritually.

Nevertheless, an even more basic question remains unanswered: How does one become motivated to seek this substitute whether it is running or some other new life-style?

George Valiant, a Harvard psychiatrist who has been studying the natural history of alcoholism, thinks he has found that answer. Alcoholics, he says, become ex-alcoholics and social drinkers through various substitutes and surrogates, but they seek that help only when they realize they have lost control of their lives.

"The key to recovery," says Valiant, "seems to be that they were no longer consciously in control of their drinking and that their use of alcohol was no longer under voluntary control." This self-discovery is a highly personal process. Unless this raising of consciousness occurs, no therapy will work. No substitute will be effective. No surrogate will take over. The addiction will continue to dominate one's life.

It is not enough, however, to stop smoking or drinking. That is an oversimplified goal. Release from bondage, however painful, says Valiant, rarely brings instant relief. Depression and divorce are common in the early stages of abstinence. The real goal is not the abstinence but a new and satisfactory existence.

In the accomplishment of this goal, there are, according to Valiant, four factors: behavior modifications, substitute dependencies, religious involvement and new relationships.

"Whoever understands human nature," wrote Sigmund Freud, "knows that hardly anything is harder for a man to give up than a pleasure he has once experienced." Freud might well have been referring to his own smoking. He was a smoker and continued to be one through thirty-three operations for cancer of the jaw and oral cavity. Apparently the father of modern psychiatry was unable to mobilize the therapeutic forces that would break the chains that bound him to this habit.

In this he has a lot in common with the common folk who

smoke. There are millions of smokers who would like to be ex-smokers. Innumerable people feeding coins into cigarette machines wish they could kick the habit. Any number of our friends and neighbors wish the day would dawn when they would not have the urge to light up just one more cigarette. Most of them have gone the route of Mark Twain, who said that giving up smoking was easy. He had done it thousands of times.

I recall an interview with the actor Dennis Hopper. He had admitted frankly as he sat there smoking a cigarette that he also smoked pot. When asked whether or not he was afraid of getting addicted to marijuana, he said absolutely not. Holding up his cigarette, he said, "It's these things that I can't get rid of."

What is the basis of the pleasure that comes from cigarettes and the subsequent habituation? What it comes down to is a dependence on nicotine. Smokers have a physical dependence on nicotine. Eventually it is not only the positive effects that keep a person smoking but the negative ones as well. What happens when smoking is stopped is too awful to contemplate. And the desire to smoke remains unchanged.

The infinite variety of methods used to break this dependence and their almost universal failure show how firmly entrenched is this need. It defeats almost every attempt to cure it. The World Health Organization defines such dependence as having physiological adaptive effects. These include (1) tolerance, (2) increased capacity to metabolize and excrete the substance, (3) withdrawal symptoms.

The withdrawal symptoms are particularly distressing, and part of that is the craving that comes about through the adaptive mechanisms in the brain and nervous system. Most of these reactions are subjective and apparent only to the victim. Depression, irritability, anxiety, restlessness and difficulty in concentrating are some of these symptoms. Others are objective and demonstrable like sweating and changes in sleep electroencephalograms, and impaired ability to perform under stressful conditions.

Both subjective and objective effects can be rapidly reversed by infusing nicotine intravenously. The same result can also be achieved simply by smoking a cigarette. It is the nicotine in the cigarette that creates dependence and relieves the symptoms of withdrawal.

Some things we know about nicotine are helpful in understanding the smoker's problem. It is a drug whose primary action is stimulation of the brain and nervous system. It also can be, in later stages, a depressant. It is even a depressant in some areas and a stimulant in others. Nicotine is rapidly absorbed. Peak levels can be obtained within minutes of lighting up a cigarette. It is also rapidly metabolized by the liver. Nicotine has a half life of 30 minutes, bringing about the cigarette-every-half-hour syndrome that most smokers have.

Usually those who persist in the habit have one or more of six reasons for doing so. These have been outlined by Dr. Daniel Horn, the former director of the National Clearing House for Smoking and Health. Those reasons are 1) stimulation 2) handling 3) pleasurable relaxation 4) crutch 5) craving 6) habit. Horn has devised a self-assessment test consisting of 18 questions which he claims can pinpoint the specific needs that are being satisfied through smoking.

Horn also listed the six most powerful motives for stopping smoking: health, expense, social influence, example, esthetics and mastery. In my own medical practice I have seen all these motives fail. Threats about health rarely work. Expense in such matters is never decisive. Segregation into a smoking section is more likely to make a smoker smoke more furiously than desist. Esthetics doesn't work even for artists. This leaves mastery, which can be a most powerful weapon. When a person finally asks, "Who is in charge here, me or the butts?" changes may occur. And if they do, these changes are quite likely to become permanent.

Nevertheless, the best guide in this therapy is still the man who couldn't give up smoking himself, Sigmund Freud. "Actually we never give anything up," he said. "We exchange one thing for another. What appears to be a renunciation is really the formation of a substitute or a surrogate."

Chapter Ten
On Assessing

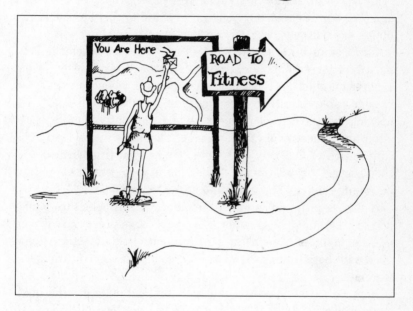

". . . . pulse can tell nonathletes just how bad things are—and how good things can be. Individuals with a pulse in the 90s are cheating themselves of an active life. Those in the 70s are settling for less than they can get. If you are in the low 60s you could be living those dreams of glory."

MANY PEOPLE ARE UNEASY beginning a fitness program. They see fitness as a high-technology industry. Articles, brochures and advertisements bombard us with the need of specialists and their special equipment. Fitness centers abound with physiologists who use sophisticated devices to test and monitor their clients. Fitness appears to be safe and sure only when we have access to the evaluations and counseling provided by such centers. The ordinary out-of-shape individual, especially those of advanced age (the ads suggest thirty-five!), is made to feel he should not undertake a fitness program without a guide.

I am reminded of those books of my youth in which the hero must face incredible odds to survive—stories about a soft, pleasure-loving dilettante marooned on a desert island, or lost in an impenetrable forest or escaping over uninhabitable land with nothing but the clothes on his back and the contents of his pockets. The outcome is always the same. The hero rapidly learns the capabilities of his body and mind. He is soon transformed into the creature he was meant to be, the few objects in his pocket becoming the only equipment he needs to survive.

A fitness program is much the same. A soft, pleasure-loving dilettante can gain confidence, survive and prosper, with no more equipment than a few common household objects. All you need as a beginner are a mirror, a scale, a tape measure and a watch.

Begin with the mirror. Undress and stand nude in front of it. Your reflection tells all. If you look fat, you are fat. You also know where that fat is. If it is on the face and the belly, it will come off readily. If it is on the hips and thighs, it will be the last to go.

Now get on the scale. It will register fat you cannot see. Match your present weight against the weight you were when you were last active and athletic. This was most likely when you graduated from college or got married. At that point, you were probably 12 percent body fat if a male, 18 percent if a female. Everything you have gained since then is fat. A very simple calculation comparing the two weights will give you a rough estimate of your current percentage of body fat.

The scale soon assumes less importance. As you become fit, muscle will replace fat. You may even gain weight, although it generally remains constant and shows no change for some months. What will change are your measurements.

Next take the tape measure and establish those measurements. Check the circumference of your calves, thighs, hips, waist and chest. As you progress, these figures will tell you about fat loss and muscle replacement. Women will often go down as much as two dress sizes while the weight remains the same.

Finally, we come to the watch. You will use this to establish your present level of fitness. This test requires one additional object. A place where you can measure how far you can go in 12 minutes. The best setting for this is usually a quarter-mile track, usually available to you at your local high school.

Warm up with a walk or a very easy jog for 10 minutes. This will raise a sweat and get you into your "second wind." Wait about five minutes, then start. Walk or walk-jog or jog at a constant speed for 12 minutes. Now stop and measure how far you have gone.

Kenneth Cooper's aerobic tables will tell you how you rate on the fitness ladder. After 8 to 12 weeks, you can repeat the test to see how much you have improved.

Predicted Maximal Oxygen Consumption on the Basis of 12-Minute Performance

Distance (miles)	Laps (¼ mile)	Max. Ox. Con. (ml/kg/min)
1.0	4	25
1.25	5	33
1.5	6	42.6
1.75	7	51.6
2.0	8	60.2

Levels of Fitness Based on 12-Minute
Performance and Maximal Oxygen Consumption

Distance (miles)	Max. Ox. Con.	Fitness level
Less than 1	Less than 25	Very poor
1–1.25	25–33	Poor
1.25–1.5	33–42	Fair
1.5–1.75	42–51	Good
1.75 or more	51 or more	Excellent

As the program progresses, your pulse rate becomes all important. It may not be quite as fixed as the North Star, but it is the best navigational guide in traveling this uncharted land. Occasional trips to the mirror, scale and tape measure will also reassure you that you are on the right track. They will help you survive your fitness program in fine style.

MY RESTING PULSE IS 48. No big deal, you might say. My resting pulse is simply part of my physical makeup. Distinctive to me but no more important than the length of my nose. My resting pulse may be slow, but that does not necessarily mean I am a superior runner. My resting pulse is, to an extent, a conversation piece. Something to drop into the discussion at the hospital lunch table or at a postrace party. It is something I possess like a condominium in Florida or a loft in Soho. Something I display much as a friend of mine wears a belt with a BMW buckle.

But this morning my pulse rate was even lower, 42 beats a minute. Six beats below normal. This is a rare treat. No matter that I don't know the physiology responsible for it; a pulse rate this low must mean great things. Just ahead are outstanding races, personal bests and feats beyond the dreams of glory.

Nonsense? Perhaps, but rightly or wrongly, runners equate their pulse rates with performance. A slow pulse rate is a runner's proudest possession. It has to do with being a runner since birth. First we are born with this capability of lowering our pulse. And then we take on the task of doing the necessary training to bring it down as far as possible. A slow pulse means that you are special. Special by birth, and special by your dedication to your sport.

My slow pulse rate does not mean I am better than another runner. It does mean that I am the best I can be. The pulse rate is, therefore, as important as runners think it is. Important physically, psychologically and spiritually. It is a numerical description of who you are, an indication of how seriously you take becoming that person.

It is an experiment anyone can perform. I once attended Grand Rounds at a midwest hospital where the medical resident presented a case study of a beginning athlete. He displayed charts showing a fall in the pulse over a period of three months, from a resting pulse of over 70 to a new level of 52.

At the end of the meeting he disclosed that he was the subject of the case. He had been assigned to conduct a meeting on the significance of the pulse rate in a fitness program and had selected himself to be the guinea pig.

This drop in the pulse rate is the almost universal result of any fitness program. Few individuals who undertake a training schedule fail to have some drop in heart rate, and sometimes the decrease can be extreme. A Finnish study of thirty-five male endurance runners using 24-hour monitoring revealed that their lowest nocturnal heart rates averaged 37 beats per minute. There has been a report in the German literature of nine runners who had resting pulses below 30, and I have had some correspondence with a Canadian marathoner whose basal pulse is 26. In such company a runner with a mediocre 48 would best remain silent.

This slow-down is usually ascribed to increased vagal influence on the heart action. The vagus nerve is part of the two-pronged autonomic nervous system that controls the heart rate. The sympathetic system speeds it up and the vagus slows it down. The relative balance between these two systems determines the rate. Training, in ways we are not sure, reduces sympathetic tone and/ or increases vagal stimulation.

Slowing of the heart rate, or bradycardia, is only one of the effects that training has on the heart rate. The same Finnish study revealed other abnormalities. One third of the athletes experienced pauses in the heart rate exceeding two seconds in length, making the immediate heart rate less than 30 per minute. Another interesting finding was the presence of first-degree heart block, a slowing of the impulse time between auricle and ventricle, in 37 percent of the athletes. More than one-fifth of them had a second-degree heart block, the Wenckebach type, with varying electrical delays resulting in intermittent dropped beats. A standard second-degree block was found in an additional 8 percent. Twenty percent had a peculiarity known as junctional rhythm, in which the beat was originating elsewhere than in the usual sinus source.

Fortunately, for most runners, these oddities mostly occur only after prolonged rest. Israeli investigators discovered this when a soccer player inadvertently was left on the examination table 45 minutes waiting for an electrocardiogram. When taken, it revealed a typical Wenckebach pattern. Subsequently, studies on other athletes using a long resting period show a significant number of abnormalities.

Such findings are the result of heavy training and represent a superior state of fitness. They should not alarm the physicians, but they do. I was once asked to examine a marine captain who had been denied clearance for the Marine Corps Marathon because of a Wenckebach heart block. When I questioned him about his training he said he ran twice a day. Six miles at lunchtime with two marine friends. Eight miles at night by himself. Then I asked him about the intensity of these workouts. His evening run, he said, was leisurely. "What about your lunch-hour runs?" I asked him. "I might be able to manage a 'yes' or a 'no,'" he answered. This man was racing six miles everyday, and then adding an hour of running at night. His EKG reflected this high degree of training. His Wenckebach was not pathological, it was physiological.

THE PULSE RATE OF IMPORTANCE is the one when you awake in the morning. Presumably that is your resting state and represents your basal metabolic rate. You are still in torpor, doing little more than idling your engine.

As soon as you get into operation your metabolism rises. Shave, shower and dress and it will have already escalated. Now comes breakfast and coffee and it increases some more. Then the movement and effort to get to work requires a higher metabolic rate. The stress there will take it even higher.

As your metabolism increases, whatever the reason, your pulse rises also. Your pulse, therefore, presents the same problem faced in doing basal metabolism tests. Preferably they are done in bed with the individual not fully awake. Simulating this situation in a person coming to a clinical laboratory is understandably difficult. The best that can be done is to have him lie down in a quiet room, make his mind a blank, and relax.

It goes without saying that once you are told to relax you tense up. Once your body knows it is going to have its pulse taken, it worries about the outcome. Adrenaline pours into your system; the pulse goes up rather than down. You must create a diversion if you are to catch your prey unaware.

How does one become indifferent to the whole pulse-taking procedure? My method is to hyperventilate. If I have forgotten to take my pulse before I get up out of bed, I take deep, slow breaths until I feel relaxed and a little light-headed. When I count my pulse, it is as if someone else were doing it. My attention is turned inward to the slow lub-dub of the heartbeat. All apprehension has vanished. Then I maintain this state until the minute is up and I get the answer.

YOU CAN ACHIEVE THE SAME EFFECT by using Benson's Relaxation Technique or some form of TM. They have been proven to produce a hypometabolic state. And that is precisely what you must be in to find out your lowest possible pulse.

It is far better, of course, to get this result before the day has begun, and to plan your life accordingly. If you are a nonathlete, this pulse rate can be a good motivator. It is not a precise statement of your level of fitness, but it does tell you roughly just where you are. It is also an indication of where you could be. Whatever your pulse, there are good reasons for doing something about it.

Should your resting pulse be in the 55–60 range, you are an out-of-shape athlete with great endurance potential. You are missing out on some particularly satisfying sports experience. A sedentary individual with a resting pulse in the 50s may well have remarkable talent for endurance events.

If your pulse is 75, you fall into the average group. This means that you are likely to be operating at a rate considerably lower than your capacity. Exercise will increase your maximum oxygen uptake as much as 25 percent and your physical work capacity as much as 300 percent.

A pulse over 90 is bad news. An Israeli study of 600 people using an equation including age, height, weight and resting-heart rate reported that those with rates in the 55–60 range had a 25 percent higher oxygen capacity than the group whose rate was 91–95.

You must interpret these numbers with caution, however. Occasionally the high pulse is due to hypermetabolism as, for instance, in a hyperthyroid state. There are also people who are hyperreactors. They can never have their pulse taken (or their blood pressure, for that matter) that it doesn't go up instantly.

Nevertheless, this baseline pulse can tell nonathletes just how bad things are—and how good things can be. Individuals with a pulse in the 90s are cheating themselves of an active life. Those in the 70s are settling for less than they can get. If you are in the low 60s you could be living those dreams of glory.

Chapter Eleven
On
Exercising

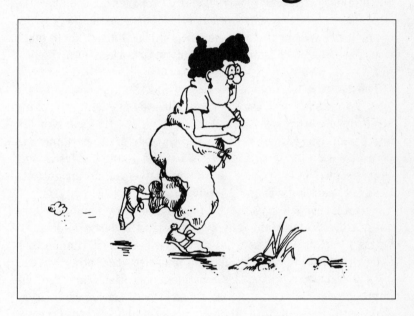

"Great legs are a great asset. Somewhere
resident in the muscles is the ability to
withstand fatigue, to handle stress and to get
the most out of your physical life. So don't
run for your heart or lungs or liver or
kidneys. Run for your muscles."

THE WOMAN on the Denver TV program was looking at a picture of me on the cover of my new book.

"You've got great legs," she said. "I'm envious. All you runners have great legs."

It's true; we do. I know I have great legs. At every race I see proof that this woman is right. Ordinary runners have extraordinary legs.

Running, whatever else it does, is apparently good for the legs. There is controversy about other parts of the body. Does running help the heart? Is it beneficial to the lungs? These questions are debated continually, not only in the press but in medical journals as well.

The benefits of running go far beyond the appearance of the legs. I do not mention the size, configuration and definition of my legs from sheer vanity—although I do not deny that this element is present. No, I bring my legs and the legs of other runners to your attention for a specific reason—to aid you in understanding exercise physiology. These legs should give you an insight into the effect running has on the body.

You might suspect from the emphasis on cardiopulmonary fitness today that training involves mostly the heart and lungs. Guess again. No matter what you have been told, running primarily trains and conditions the muscles; the other organs merely assist in realizing this functional potential. Almost all the improvement in performance occurs because of circulatory changes in the muscles and changes in the muscle cells, the engines that transform chemical energy into mechanical energy.

We had no idea of the magnitude of such changes until the late 1960s, when muscle biopsy techniques came into general use. We then discovered an increase in the number of capillaries supplying blood to the muscles, an expanded ability of muscles to extract oxygen from the blood, and more metabolism-controlling enzymes in the muscle cells of active people. All of these improve physical work capacity. My leg muscles and yours can, with minimal change in the heart, do as much as 300 percent more work —which is why people with greatly damaged hearts can train up to the marathon level.

Cardiac rehabilitation, therefore, is mainly *muscle* rehabilitation. Heart patients conquer fatigue by developing great legs.

Physiologist Gordon Cumming points out, "The peripheral circulation regulation and the improvement in the metabolic processes in the muscle can account for the improvement in endurance performance in the absence of an increase in heart-stroke volume."

Dr. John Holloszy, a pioneer in this work, agrees with Cumming. "It seems unlikely," he states, "that cardiac adaptations play a role in protection against skeletal fatigue."

I have been a physician for 40 years and a runner for 18, yet this was news to me. I now realize that I never quite understood what was going on. I studied running and performance all those years and never got the hang of it.

If runners have great legs, and they obviously do, it means that fitness programs have to do with leg muscles rather than the heart muscle. The emphasis in training, therefore, ought to be on "perceived exertion"—what the body feels. Forget about heart rates and focus on training your legs.

You can see, too, that *whatever ails you, a potentially trainable pair of legs is all you need to embark upon a fitness program.* Should you have bad lungs or a bad heart, diabetes or hypertension, obesity or colitis, arthritis or depression, you can still develop great legs—and also your full functional potential.

Medical sages seem to know this. Before physicians became caught up in the technology of disease, they realized the importance of muscle tone. When the late cardiologist Paul Dudley White was called upon to assess a patient's capacity to withstand surgery, it was his custom to examine the legs. If they were firm and well muscled, he would give his approval.

Great legs are a great asset. Somewhere resident in the muscles is the ability to withstand fatigue, to handle stress and to get the most out of your physical life. So don't run for your heart or lungs or liver or kidneys. Run for your muscles. It makes more sense.

WHEN YOU TRAIN three things happen to your muscles and two of them are bad. The prime movers, the power muscles, become short and inflexible. The antagonist muscles that modulate the action become relatively weak. This strength/flexibility imbalance causes or is a major contributor to injuries in our various sports.

When a person is involved in a sport that demands thousands of repetitions of a particular movement these imbalances are bound to occur. Training of the legs, for instance, results in development of the muscles of the back of the leg, the thigh and the low back. At the same time muscles of the shins, front thighs, the abdomen and the buttocks become relatively weak.

These postural weaknesses put abnormal stress on the foot, leg, knee, thigh and low back. A variety of overuse syndromes can then occur. This is especially true if there is some associated structural weakness.

The short, powerful calf muscle combines with weak shin muscle in contributing to such injuries as shinsplints, Achilles tendinitis, plantar fasciitis and calf cramps.

The muscle imbalance from the knee up causes malposition of the pelvis and a host of problems involving the low back, sciatic nerves and hip joints.

Prevention is best accomplished by regular remedial exercises. The three muscles on the back side of the body must be stretched. The three opposing muscle groups on the front of the body must be strengthened.

The stretching is easily described and appears quite simple but must be done with great care. At no time should there be pain or discomfort, the limiting point should be simply a feeling of tension.

The first exercise is performed standing an arm's length away from the wall with feet flat on the floor. Lean forward until your chest is against the wall, feet still flat and the body forming a straight line from heel to chest. Hold for 10 seconds. Then return to upright. Repeat 10 times.

The second stretch consists of standing on one leg, knee locked, and placing the other straight leg (knee locked) on a step, stool or table depending on your level of flexibility. Attempt to touch your head to your knee—you may achieve only an approximation. Again do not go beyond feeling of tension. Hold for 10 seconds then return to upright. Repeat 10 times.

The final stretch is the backover. Lie on your back on the ground, legs out straight, knees locked. Bring legs over your head toward the floor behind it. Touch floor if possible, but under no circumstances go beyond the feeling of tension. Hold for 10 seconds then return to resting state. Repeat 10 times.

The strengthening exercises involve the opposing muscles. The first two use weights of five pounds to ten pounds (or a paint can with water). Sit on the edge of a table and place the weight over the foot. Now flex the foot upward, keeping the leg immobile. Hold for 10 seconds. Relax. Repeat 10 times.

Next, still sitting on the table and using the same weights on the foot, straighten the leg and lock the knee. Hold for 10 seconds. Relax. Repeat 10 times.

The final exercise is the bent-leg situp. Lie on your back with your knees bent and your feet flat on the floor. Now tighten your buttocks and bring your head and upper chest to a 45-degree angle off the floor. Hold for 10 seconds. Relax. Repeat 10 times. Have someone hold your feet or lock them under a chair, if necessary.

Done on a daily basis, these small groups of exercises will provide considerable protection against the injuries that beset athletes. When injury does occur, they should be used in conjunction with other forms of therapy.

AT THOSE TIMES in the past when I viewed the body as a machine rather than a function of the unified self, I pictured the heart as the engine. The heart is all noise and movement, with an independent existence. It idles even when I am at rest, and when I exert myself it dominates my senses. I can feel and hear it; I can even see it on the EKG monitor during my stress test.

But the heart, for all its evident activity, is not my engine. The muscle is. It is the individual muscle cell, joined with thousands of others, that makes my body go. The individual muscle cell is the engine that changes chemical energy into physical energy. It extracts oxygen from the blood and uses it, stores up sugar and then burns it, takes in fats and triglycerides and converts them into power. The muscle cell uses protein to manufacture the mitochondria that take up the oxygen, and it produces the enzymes that control most of the miraculous metabolic events that occur in our bodies.

By comparison, the heart does little. It is true that the heart muscle, the myocardium, enlarges with activity; true also that the cardiac output is increased. The efficiency of the heart improves. The heart becomes capable of more work. But none of the other metabolic marvels takes place. The myocardium shows no change in mitochondria, no increase in enzymes. The heart, you see, is not the engine; it is no more than a fuel pump.

The heart brings the necessary fuel to the muscle cell—the oxygen from the lungs, the food processed by the gastrointestinal tract. The muscle does the rest. More than 90 percent of our calories are burned by muscle.

When I exercise, the heart is affected only secondarily. The primary effect is on the muscle mass that is being used. It is the muscle that uses up the calories and reduces my weight. It is the muscle that removes the cholesterol and triglycerides and gives me a good lipid profile. It is the muscle that would reduce the need for insulin were I a diabetic. It is the efficiency of the muscle that allows the cardiac patient to do more work. It is the improved function of this engine that conquers fatigue.

That is why I am the best getting better when I run. Effort breeds effort. Mileage makes for more mileage. The engine does more with less. I have gotten so I can almost feel it all happening: the capillaries multiplying, the mitochondria enlarging, the enzymes increasing. I am propelled by this fantastic engine whose operation is one of the wonders of the world.

I can see why I thought it was the heart that did all those things. The term "aerobic exercise," for one thing. It is scientifically correct; the muscle performs best with an adequate supply of oxygen. But the word "aerobic" made me think of heart and lungs. It emphasizes the organs that supply the oxygen, not the muscle that uses it.

So too with the stated goal of "cardiopulmonary fitness." It is evident now that the primary aim of an exercise program is *muscular* fitness. One becomes an athlete because of the athletic things that are happening in the muscle.

Another major distraction has been the use of maximal oxygen uptake as the best measure of fitness. Not only does the name suggest that the heart and lungs are the organs at issue, but the test result actually changes very little with major improvements in fitness. Maximal oxygen uptake operates within limits preset by heredity. We can ordinarily improve it by only about 20 percent.

The indicator of physical fitness is physical work capacity. This is the ability to do submaximal work to exhaustion. My physical work capacity is entirely a matter of how good my engine muscle is. While my maximal oxygen capacity can only increase 20 percent on my running program, my physical work capacity can increase by as much as *300 percent*.

Knowing what is happening when I run has had a liberating effect on me. There is no need to use target heart rates. If the muscle is being trained, not the heart, why monitor my pulse? I listen to my body and react accordingly. When I train, I ask my muscle for a pace that I can hold indefinitely. I dial my body to "comfortable"—not too easy, not too hard—then hold it there, knowing that pace will accomplish all the physiological and bio-chemical events needed for fitness.

This ability of my body to know what it is doing is called "perceived exertion." It is the most liberating discovery an individual can make. I no longer need charts or graphs; all I need is my river road and some free time. Further, there has been scientific confirmation of my own experience.

"Perception of effort," states sports psychologist William Morgan, "is directly related to exertional cost in 90 percent of all the subjects tested. It is a perfect linear function."

Now I understand why my running is getting better. My muscles are functioning better and better. Athletes the world over have known that it is the legs that go first, not the heart, as the medical profession seems to believe. Athletes equate performance and fitness with the legs. That's the way it is on the run.

I HAD COME TO DALLAS to champion the cause of physical exercise for patients with lung disease. I was at the respiratory therapists' annual meeting to deliver the usual message: "Treat the whole patient." Specialists tend to forget this. They forget that disease is only part of the problem, and that they must treat the patient's illness and predicament as well.

Disease is a biological process. Illness is the impact that disease has on a patient's life. The predicament is the psychosocial situation in which the patient lives. There are instances where the disease may not be improved in any way, yet treating the illness and the patient's life situation can give almost miraculous results.

Specialists—and these respiratory therapists were specialists —know too much about disease and too little about health; too much about the limitations of the body and too little about its potential; too much about what goes on in their primary interest (in this case the lungs) and too little about what goes on in the rest of the body.

Just before my talk in Dallas I had taken a tour of the convention floor. One booth after another displayed machines and devices designed for new and better ways to diagnose and treat pulmonary disease. One instrument could take ordinary air in your house and change it into 95 percent oxygen. When I took a deep breath, another converted it into a computer printout with a half-dozen tests and graphs of my exhalation.

Now I was on the podium asking the therapists to turn their backs for a moment on all this shiny equipment. I wanted them to discard their specialist mentalities about the human body. For my allotted minutes, I wanted to be talking to generalists who saw that everything was connected to something else.

The lungs, I told them, do not exist in a vacuum. In real life they are connected to the heart, and the heart to the circulatory system, and the circulatory system to the muscles. Anatomy does not begin and end with the bronchopulmonary tree.

This holistic approach to the patient is extremely important in lung disease. Without it, the therapist may not understand the use of exercise in treatment. Exercise, you should know, has a bad name among the pulmonary specialists, because it does not improve pulmonary function. Study upon study has shown that.

"Breathing exercises and similar gymnastics performed under controlled conditions," reported one investigator, "have no substantial effect on ventilatory capacity and blood-gas tensions in groups of patients with obstructive pulmonary disease." This investigator went on to suggest that any improvement that occurs is psychological and due to the enthusiasm of the physician.

I looked out on the therapists and went immediately to the attack. I conceded that pulmonary-function tests don't change. Forget about these tests, I told them. Learn exercise physiology. Learn that the adaptation to exercise occurs mainly at the level of the heart, the circulatory system and the muscles. The lungs deliver the oxygen, it's true, but the heart and muscles can learn to use it more efficiently.

The factors that influence our aerobic capacity are mostly circulatory and muscular, regardless of lung capacity. Indeed, even when the heart cannot improve, the changes at the muscular level can result in major improvements in aerobic capacity. Bengt Saltin, the Danish exercise physiologist, has made this point repeatedly.

"Increases in maximal aerobic power that accompany physical conditioning," he writes, "are predominantly due to increased muscle blood flow and muscle capillary density."

Get rid of your old ideas about the lungs, I told the therapists. They are not all-important. The lungs, I said, are no more than the gas tank. They take in the gas, which is oxygen. When you have a patient with lung disease, that gas tank is smaller. That makes things difficult but not impossible. The logical thing to do is to increase the efficiency of the car and engine so that you can get farther on that gas.

That is what exercise does. First it streamlines the body by lessening the percentage of body fat. Then it delivers more oxygen through an increase in blood volume and an increase in capillaries in the muscle tissue. The heart pump is improved, so all of this takes place more easily. And when this oxygen is sent to the muscle, more of it is taken up. Studies have shown that the difference between the oxygen going in to muscle and the oxygen in the veins coming out of the muscle is increased.

These are things none of the technology in the convention hall could do. What was needed was a solid understanding of exercise physiology. Then these specialists could treat patients with an air of confidence in an atmosphere filled with optimism. Enthusiasm always helps, but it also helps if you understand what you are doing. It is not enough to determine to treat the whole patient. You must first learn how that whole patient works.

Chapter Twelve
On Energizing

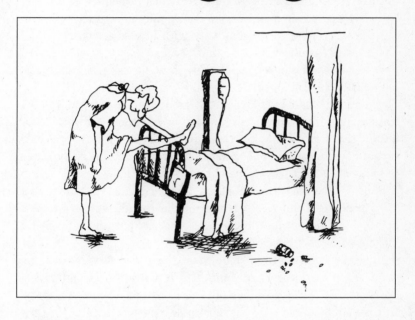

"There is a healthy way to be ill. Improving physical work capacity will also improve the capacity to deal with any disease. Whatever the disease, a patient can always use increased energy and vitality. Well-trained muscles can compensate for handicaps in other systems."

"HAVE YOU NOTICED," asked the man at the Boston airport, "that there is one place where there are never fitness programs?"

This man was an expert on fitness, a runner who had turned his avocation into a livelihood. He had run the marathon the previous day and was now returning to California, where he headed a firm that set up fitness programs for corporations.

I also am an expert on fitness. At times, it seems that all my time is occupied by fitness. I am continually in contact with people who are engaged in some way with fitness activities. But I had no ready reply to his question.

When I asked where this place with no fitness programs was, he answered, "The hospitals."

I knew he was right. Except for an occasional cardiac rehabilitation unit, most hospitals do not have fitness programs for either their personnel or their patients. Aerobic exercise is rarely used in a hospital setting. Seldom is a patient encouraged to make the effort to become fit.

Shortly after that conversation, I learned this truth firsthand. I injured a calf muscle and was unable to run, so I went to a hospital physiotherapy department to work out on the exercise bicycle while the muscle healed.

I had not been there in some time. For the last two years, my medical chores have been limited to reading EKGs and giving stress tests. I no longer manage the day-to-day care of patients, so I have no occasion to visit most of the hospital.

The physiotherapy department was twice as big as I remembered it and filled with a variety of new electrical machines. In almost every booth, there was a patient being treated passively on a table. In the midst of this impressive professional activity was the one exercise bike, an ancient cast-iron monster called the "Everlast."

I mounted the bike and pedaled furiously for about 30 minutes. When I finished, a therapist came over to me.

"Doc," he said, "you are the first one to use that bike in two years."

The one training machine in the department, the mainstay of

any fitness program for the diseased or handicapped, had not been used in all that time.

"The last one to use it," he said, "was Felix."

I remembered Felix. He had been my patient. His chronic lung ailment made him short of breath at rest, and he could hardly make it from the bed to the bathroom. Felix was in and out of the hospital like a yo-yo. When I sent for his old records, I was told they might have to be brought in with a cart. Felix was a constant problem for himself and his doctors.

One day, it occurred to me that training might help him. Before I began running, I was out of breath after running 100 yards. My improvement in endurance was not due to my lungs. My vital capacity, always high-normal, had never changed—but my fitness had. Perhaps Felix could improve without changing his lung function.

"Felix," I told him, "you are going to PT tomorrow and pedal that exercise bike until you're exhausted. And you'll do that every day until you go home."

He did, and the change was remarkable. He still wheezed at rest, but his walking improved tremendously. Felix left feeling better than he had in years.

He came back to the hospital, of course. When he got home, he just sat around. You cannot put fitness in the bank; you have to earn it every day. So Felix returned for treatment—but at longer intervals than before, and he stayed for shorter times. During each subsequent admission, he rode the bike daily.

Now nobody rides the bike. No patient in this 600-bed hospital is training for endurance. No one is working for maximal physical function, no physician is employing physiology in the treatment of disease, no physician is treating the whole patient.

Nor am I to be excused. When I left my practice, I forgot about Felix and the bike. It had been a one-time thing, and he had been the only patient I'd ever sent to the bike. It did not occur to me then that there was a major role for fitness in the hospital.

WHEN YOU HEAR that the only exercise bike in a busy hospital physiotherapy department has not been used in two years, you begin to wonder. Why is it that hospitals do not have fitness programs? Why don't physicians urge patients to use exercise as well as medicine? Why do health-care professionals appear unconvinced of the value of physical training in the treatment of diseases?

For quite good reasons: Physicians, however little they know about exercise physiology, know a great deal about disease. They treat it daily and they study it constantly. They are suspicious of any therapies that arise outside their orthodoxy. Their tendency is to regard people outside their ranks as pushy promoters of their own interests. They demand solid scientific proof for claims of benefits for any new treatment—including exercise.

That scientific proof is not forthcoming. Physicians therefore have a tendency to see fitness as a media event with little substance. Their noncompliance indicates a basic distrust of the fitness premise, and their reading confirms that suspicion. "There is no definitive evidence," states Dr. Victor Froehlicker, a prominent heart researcher, "that exercise is effective in the primary or secondary or tertiary prevention of coronary heart disease."

Even the proselytizers for fitness acknowledge this observation. Should you listen to the leaders of the fitness movement you would find the talks are larded with qualifying words and phrases. Preceding each claim is a "may" or a "might" or a "should." The effects of exercise on disease remain speculative, and medicine is not a speculative sport.

Physicians know enough about the inexorable progression of disease to doubt that there are any lasting effects from exercise. They know pathology. They do not believe that disease can be altered simply by body movement. Theirs is a profession of skeptics and cynics. They deal in pain and suffering and death. The optimistic promises of the proponents of running and other exercise turn them off rather than on.

This suspicion even includes cardiac rehabilitation, the one program that seems to have caught on in hospitals. Even in cardiac rehab, the doctors are dragging their feet. Most patients are self-referred. They have taken it upon themselves to enter these programs, frequently against the advice of their physicians or at best with their reluctant consent.

But here, too, the doctors are on fairly solid ground. A recent review of all the available work on exercise and heart disease came to the same conclusion. According to Dr. Ezra Amsterdam, in an article in *American Heart Journal*, an exercise program will have no effect on the diseased heart. All the changes occur in the periphery, in the capillaries and the muscles.

"Numerous studies," wrote Amsterdam, "have failed to identify a direct cardiac mechanism in association with improved functional capacity following exercise training in coronary patients." That improvement occurs without cardiac improvement.

Exercise can induce the trained state regardless of disease. Every patient can be made fit. And that fitness will result in increased physical work capacity, increased oxygen intake, and reduced stress on the heart. Again it is understandable that physicians have been unaware of this. In the average American medical school only four hours in the four-year curriculum are spent on the effect of exercise on the body.

So there it is. Exercise programs have gained no foothold in hospitals for two reasons: The doctors know too much about disease and too little about exercise physiology. They rightly say there is no evidence that disease is in any way influenced by exercise. But they know so little physiology that they are unaware how exercise will profit every patient regardless of the disease.

There is a healthy way to be ill. Improving physical work capacity will also improve the capacity to deal with any disease. Whatever the disease, a patient can always use increased energy and vitality. Well-trained muscles can compensate for handicaps in other systems.

Physicians have yet to elevate their consciousness about these capabilities in their patients—and about their own opportunities to develop them. Hospital patients follow orders. They can be sent to physiotherapy, told to pedal to exhaustion, made to become fit. Physicians frustrated by their patients' not following negative injunctions such as "Stop smoking," "Stop drinking," "Stop overeating" can induce them to do something positive for their health.

Doctors have been told from their first year in medical school to treat the whole patient. They just have never been taught how. Once physicians learn the basics of exercise physiology, they will be able to offer total care—and then fitness programs will become routine in our hospitals.

WHAT HAS EXERCISE TO OFFER? Not prevention of heart disease. Dr. Froehlicker has told us that there is no evidence that exercise is effective in the primary, secondary or tertiary prevention of coronary heart disease. Nor does exercise offer improvement for an existing disease. Dr. Amsterdam, in reviewing the available research, could not find proof that there were any direct cardiac effects of training in coronary patients.

What exercise has to offer is the attainment of maximal work capacity. Exercise will bring any individual to a trained state. Many medical reports speak of the "subjective" benefits associated with regular exercise, as if they were all in the person's mind. They are not. These results are quite objective and scientific. They can be easily tested on a bicycle or treadmill.

The limitations of disease on physical work capacity are much less than we suspect. The capabilities of handicapped people, whatever the handicap, are truly amazing. Wherever the possibilities of fitness are explored, a life is changed. There is the birth of a new capability, a new spirit, a new future.

Exercise physiology is the health science that will bring that capability, that spirit and that future to medicine. We need an exercise physiologist as part of the health care team. There should be one in every hospital, one available for consultation for every patient on the way to recovery and a new life.

ONE OF THE BEST-KNOWN cardiac rehabilitation units in the country is now accepting patients with diabetes. I have been notified by the University of Wisconsin at La Crosse that its rehabilitation unit is ready to treat physician-referred diabetics.

We are making progress. Cardiac rehabilitation is too valuable to be limited to cardiacs. Soon it will be available to all patients regardless of their disease. And not merely because exercise is good for the disease (which is still a question), but because it is good for the patient.

Exercise may be good for diabetes; it is even better for diabetics. Exercise may be good for hypertension; it is even better for hypertensives. Exercise may be good for asthma; it is even better for asthmatics. And so it goes. *Exercise may be good for a variety of diseases; it is even better for patients that have them.*

We are becoming aware of the immediate benefit of exercise on a number of diseases. We remain uncertain, however, as to whether the final prognoses of these diseases is changed in any way by exercise—whether, in fact, it will prolong a patient's life. What we do know is that exercise can prolong a patient's day. It can fill it with movement and stamina and endurance.

Exercise makes you fit—no more, no less. Fitness is the ability to do work—no more, no less. Fitness does not prevent disease; it does not cure disease. Fitness enables the body to function at a higher level. It makes people athletes, regardless of their ailment.

Once you realize that fitness is the ability to do work, a very confusing subject is clarified. Fitness becomes much easier to understand, as do the conflicts and arguments about it. If fitness is the ability to do work, there are many things fitness is not. Chiefly it has nothing to do with disease.

What fitness does is enable the diseased body to do more work —to push back the barriers of fatigue, exhaustion, shortness of breath, pain, or whatever it is that limits work. When a person with a disease becomes fit, work becomes possible, not because the disease is changed in any way, but because the working capacity of the body has been improved.

Physicians have been slow to understand this. Even the cardiologists who use exercise do it for the wrong reasons. Their target is the disease, not the patient. Other specialists have not even gotten that far. They do not see the life-giving and liberating effects of exercise. They focus on the pathology of the body.

These physicians argue that exercise will not help disease. They say there is no conclusive proof that training the body will cure or prevent most illnesses. A friend of mine who has written a text on preventive medicine once made that point quite clearly.

"George," he said, "if you show me that exercise prevents disease, I will add a chapter on it in my book." I never have, and he never will.

Exercise does not prevent anything. It adds to life, liberty and the pursuit of happiness. It is the way to achieve maximum function. Therefore, it is separate from disease. What it changes is the patient's life. Yet the very people whose lives are most affected by poor conditioning are being ignored. The people who need fitness most are being deprived of it.

"Deprived" may be too harsh a word, but I think not. These patients are locked into a diminished existence when they are unfit. Yet we doctors permit this to happen routinely. We restrict lives instead of expanding them. We narrow horizons instead of widening them. We reduce expectations instead of raising them.

We doctors are too concerned with disease and death. I share in that feeling of guilt we all have when we cannot prevent patients from dying. But I believe we should experience even more guilt because we prevent patients from *living*. We fear malpractice because our patients will die, which is in any case inevitable. We are actually guilty of malpractice when our patients are not taught to live.

Nevertheless, that is the current state of medicine. Even where there are cardiac rehabilitation programs, many of the patients are self-referred. Doctors see no need for such sweaty exuberances. Nor is the situation helped by the claims of the physicians who conduct such facilities. They should cease arguing that exercise helps cure a disease. They should take to high ground and tell us what exercise does for people: the decrease of fatigue, the increase in energy, the measurable improvement in physical work capacity, the enhancement of self-image.

All fitness needs in its support are the facts. What can be proven is enough. Athletes seek the ability to perform well. Cardiacs and hypertensives and diabetics and asthmatics and all those who have chronic diseases seek the same thing. Exercise will give it to them.

Chapter Thirteen
On Doctoring

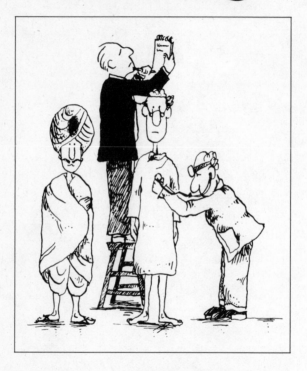

"The doctor traditionally has been a teacher. Being a coach and a motivator is not a new role. It is simply one that has fallen into disuse. Taking on that responsibility does, however, entail becoming an athlete oneself. If doctors want to open a new world of physical activity, it must be their world also."

WHEN DEALING WITH ACUTE ILLNESS, many physicians are superb. Our medical technology, the science of medical care, has outstripped the imagination. We read almost daily of new triumphs in the diagnosis and treatment of life-threatening disease. Every sizable hospital has physicians and technicians and machines capable of accomplishing miracles at a moment's notice.

Where doctors fail is in the treatment of chronic disease. The impressive victories won over acute illnesses are not duplicated in dealing with protracted and lifelong sickness. Such situations come down to getting the most out of what the patient has. This is hard work for both the physician and the patient, and neither seems up to it. The marvelous new technology in the laboratory and the mind-boggling devices in radiology are of little use. The new drugs are irrelevant. The information dispensed in medical journals and at conventions is of no help. This is a bare knuckles fight with an unforgiving opponent.

This therapeutic impasse has led to a search for alternative types of medical care, and the development of what is now called holistic medicine. The concept of holistic medicine is on the side of the angels. It is also on the side of the philosophers and the exercise physiologists. Its principles are simple, direct and on the mark.

The word "holistic," which is derived from the Greek word *holos*, or whole, was introduced by Jan Smuts, former prime minister of South Africa, in 1926. He took the position that things in this world tended to aggregate and form wholes. But holism is actually an ancient idea. We have heard it echoed down the centuries. Man is a whole, a unity or body-mind-spirit. And the whole is greater than the sum of the parts.

Holism is the basis of the concept of synergy. Things work better than seems possible when each part profits from what happens. Ruth Benedict pointed out this principle in primitive societies. Buckminster Fuller extended it to all sorts of physical and human equations. When the union occurs, two plus two equals five. An unpredictably beneficial result follows.

Predictably, holistic medicine has been accepted by those who believe that two plus two can equal five. Those individuals who

are trying to get the most out of themselves. Those more interested in performance than disease. Holistic medicine speaks to
those who believe in themselves and have faith in the universe,
those who know that they are born to be a success and there is a
way to do it—the athletes.

With more and more people wanting to be athletes, the influence of holistic medicine is widening. Now people with chronic
disease want to test their limits and act like healthy human
beings. Many are turning to the rules and regulations set up by
holistic practitioners.

"The major therapeutic emphasis of the holistic physician,"
says Dr. C. Norman Shealy, president of the American Holistic
Medical Association, "is on teaching proper life-style, nutrition,
adequate physical exercise and self-regulation techniques."

This sounds suspiciously like Hippocrates. And reading holistic tracts will reinforce that feeling. Attending a holistic medicine
convention will give you a sense that there is little progress
being made in medicine. The lectures are on procedures and
techniques that go back over the ages. The talks could easily
have been given a century ago. It is as if nothing has happened
since.

And to some extent this is quite true. We are still dealing with
the same body, the same human nature, the same chronic day-
to-day problems of body-mind-spirit. We are still occupied with
getting the most out of ourselves and our lives. The difference is
that now we have the time and the money and the ego to do it.

When ordinary medicine fails to help, people will look to some
alternative. Holistic medicine is certainly an attractive one. It
rests on a solid base of philosophy and physiology. It takes notice
of human nature. Holistic medicine subscribes to the reality principle. You are responsible for your own destiny. You control
your fate. You are the only obstacle to your perfection.

HOLISTIC MEDICINE is a wonderful idea—on paper. It has the
highest of goals, the purest of motives. It is the party of reform
with the support of tradition.

The principles of holistic medicine read like an emancipation proclamation for the patient. Its emphasis is on prevention and self-help. The patient is a participant in whatever takes place. The holistic approach recognizes that illness is caused and maintained by an interaction of biological, psychological and social forces. On paper, holistic medicine is perfect.

In actuality, holistic medicine is like a giant flea market. Anyone can set up a table and vend his or her wares. The offerings range from pure science to far-out fantasies about the body-mind-spirit integration. And each is given equal standing. Dietary pronouncements with no proof whatsoever have the same status as the confirmed truths of exercise physiology. Therapies revealed to some mystic on a mountain receive the same attention as that given to those backed by painstaking scientific research.

In holistic medicine, conjectures become truths, hypotheses become facts, theories become axioms. Simply saying something makes it true. If said enough times, it becomes holy scripture.

These are not reformers; these are revolutionaries—each with a different cause, each with a different loyalty, each with a different path to salvation. The holistic medicine movement has generated, it is true, new ways for promoting health and treating disease. It has also regenerated the bizarre human-potential movements of past decades. Ideas and practices that began with Esalen are back.

This does not sit well with orthodox physicians. The practice of medicine, no matter what else it is, must be based on scientific grounds. Doctors may use therapies that work even though they don't know why they are effective. But even in such instances, they demand proof that the treatment does what it claims to do. Such evidence is absent in many of the prescriptions of holistic practitioners. For this reason, the medical establishment has a healthy distrust of what goes on under the banner of holism.

"For some people," writes psychologist Roger Zimmerman, "holistic medicine conjures up visions of orange-colored Zen robes, herbal teas, mantras, radical vegetarian diets, and last, but not least, the entire state of California."

Zimmerman's point: Support the concept, but stay away from the words "holistic medicine."

Dr. A. J. Lipowski, a prominent psychiatrist, takes the same view. In an article tracing the holistic-medical foundations of American psychiatry, Lipowski comments on this current movement: "Holistic medicine emerged as a catchword for an anti-scientific and anti-medical approach to health and disease. This perverted use of the term must not be confused with its traditional meaning."

The people who support the new holism have captured the best words. Their brochures are a delight to the eye and the mind and the spirit. They speak of human function, of biomedical synergistics, of the inner and outer environment, of frontiers of the mind and the body, of nutrition for performance. Everything, they say, is connected with everything else. Nothing is too trivial for their attention. What is done every moment of the day impacts on the health and fitness of the individual.

These are indeed areas that orthodox medical practitioners generally ignore—or, at best, give only passing attention. These are concerns that should be part of the traditional practice of medicine but unfortunately are not.

The supporters of holism have concentrated on the traditional concerns of treating the whole person but have ignored the equally traditional standards of science in this treatment. Our present medical establishment, on the other hand, has allowed the scientific approach to dominate medicine.

"The weight of evidence suggests," says J. Ralph Audi of the University of California Medical School in San Francisco, "that the health status of the population is not largely dependent on the quantity and quality of medical care, but the ecology (lifestyle in its broadest sense) is the primary determinant."

This means that we the people are in control of our health. Our task is to take "holistic medicine"—a perfect idea, on paper— and make it a reality.

I FREQUENTLY RECEIVE LETTERS from runners in college who are preparing for medical school or one of the health-care specialties. They are interested, they tell me, in practicing some form of sports medicine. Some are worried that the medicine practiced today is too interested in disease and not enough in health. Their participation in running has changed their attitude toward the traditional view on what is normal. They want to treat the whole patient—and they prefer that the patient be an athlete.

In the past, when people asked me about practicing sports medicine, I said, "There are just not enough athletes to make a practice out of treating them."

There is no actual specialty of sports medicine. Only the orthopedic surgeons see enough athletes to make their care and treatment a paying proposition. Only in extraordinary situations can a physician survive seeing only athletes as patients.

Dr. Gabe Mirkin, a prominent writer on sports medicine, agrees. "I keep my allergy and dermatology practice," says Mirkin, "because sports medicine doesn't pay."

Only recently did it occur to me that it is possible for any doctor to practice sports medicine. It is, in fact, possible for any health-care specialist—nurse, nutritionist, physiotherapist or physiologist—to survive solely on sports medicine.

The solution: Turn the problem around. If there are not enough athletes who are patients, why not make every patient an athlete? Without changing the outward appearance of the practice, every physician could then become a sports physician.

Impossible, you might say. The tired housewife an athlete? The little old lady in tennis shoes? The cardiac, the asthmatic, the manic depressive, the alcoholic, the hypochondriac?

Why not? Think of how interesting those office hours would become. Treating the never-ending cycle of backache, constipation, headache and hypertension could become a delight. This approach could turn that dreary succession of patients into athletes a coach could be proud of.

The doctor traditionally has been a teacher. Being a coach and a motivator is not a new role. It is simply one that has fallen into disuse. Taking on that responsibility does, however, entail becoming an athlete oneself. If doctors want to open a new world of physical activity, it must be their world also.

They will need some new tools: a knowledge of exercise physiology, a grasp of the essentials of muscle function, some insight into the mysteries of rest and relaxation, a thorough knowledge of nutrition, continuing study of the effects of exercise on disease, and, finally, an awareness that there are exercise-induced diseases as well.

The runners who write to me have a head start. They know you don't have to be a motor genius to be an athlete; all you need is the desire. They know that normal is not average; it is the best you can be. And aging, they are beginning to realize, is more often than not a matter of rusting out. Deterioration sets in the day you stop moving.

There is still room in medicine for the new technology, the advances in medical science. When patients become athletes, they require the best of everything—the science as well as the art, holistic medicine in its widest meaning.

Practice sports medicine? The doctor should be practicing it every moment of every day.

Chapter Fourteen
On
Working

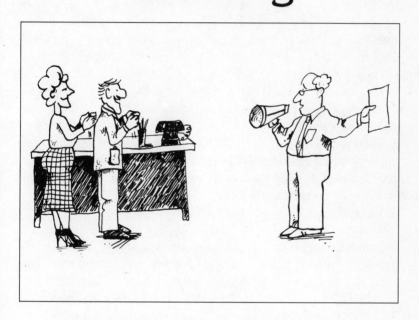

"What health is to the individual, morale is to the corporation."

THE IBM MAN and I were sitting in the lobby of a Miami Beach hotel having the "jogger's breakfast" while waiting for the IBM award convention to start. I was there to lecture on the rewards of fitness. My job: to tell the 700 award winners of the values that come with an exercise program. My function: to motivate the best to get better.

My companion was in the IBM uniform, the suit and shirt and tie. He was wearing the corporate equivalent of the pin stripes of the New York Yankees. He was on a winning team and he knew it. His interest was not in fitness, however; it was in morale.

Once morale improves, he said, so does everything else. The rest is science and technology, never a problem at IBM. Morale is the key to the successful unit, the successful division, the successful corporation.

He was the head of a new facility in the Midwest and had gone through some problems with morale. His people were all transplants. They had come not only from other geographic areas but from other departments of the company as well. Many had been in work clothes and were now in the traditional shirt and tie.

It had been a big change, and people don't take well to change. Morale had suffered. Now, however, it was on the upswing. The plant was in a small town, a good community. People were getting involved in activities within the company and in their neighborhoods. Testing had shown marked improvement in morale. The IBM man looked pleased. His morale was quite high.

It struck me then that I had come to talk about fitness without knowing what corporations really needed. I had come with an answer without knowing the question. I had focused on my specialty and saw it as the solution to everyone's difficulty. Whatever ailed American corporations could be put to rights by fitness programs. When I preached fitness I always implied that these programs would develop enthusiastic, energetic, creative employees, and I assumed that the outcome would be enthusiastic, energetic, creative corporations. I had never considered the importance of morale.

I got up then and put in a call to my newspaper in New Jersey.

I asked one of the editors to read me Webster's definition of morale. When she did, I knew the question management was asking. "Why is it that the best workers in the world, using the best technology in the world, are performing so poorly?" And I also knew the answer: "Lack of morale."

Morale, Webster tells us, is a confident, resolute, willing, courageous, self-sacrificing attitude toward a function or task demanded of an individual by a group. It is based on pride of achievement, faith in the leadership and its ultimate success, a sense of fruitful participation, and devotion and loyalty to other members.

"Morale" is one of those wonderful words the French have given us. I could almost hear the "Marseillaise" rising to a crescendo behind the voice on the phone. Morale is the quality we need for major incitements, for great deeds, and for difficult goals that require a long-term commitment.

Individual morale, according to Webster, is a state of psychological well-being and buoyancy based on such factors as mental and physical health, a sense of purpose and usefulness, and confidence in the future.

From this description, I could see that morale was of tremendous importance. Both for the individual and for the group. You could make a conscript army fit, but you would not have morale. Morale is cooperative determination, the desire to work in a common cause. Achieving good morale is the most difficult task of any leader.

Coaches know this all too well. George Allen, who transformed his over-the-hill Redskins into the best fourth-quarter team in football, said the hardest of his seven rules to put into effect was "work together." The others—work hard; improve every day; have a positive attitude; do not complain; know that no one can beat you but yourself; and, ask yourself how badly do you want it—were in comparison all easy to attain.

I remembered a statement by the coach of the Vancouver Canucks, a hockey team that had come from nowhere to get into the Stanley Cup finals. "When I took over," he said, "we had good players but a bad team. The players were totally motivated as individuals but not as a team. There was jealousy and envy. Players bragging about their success, laughing at other players." Then he brought in several young players and with them a new spirit and a winning team.

Fitness, I realized, is only part of the formula. The secret ingredient is morale. That is what motivates the best to get better. You have to be fit, but you also have to love what you do and the people you do it with.

The IBM man had left for the meeting. I followed him, eager to tell those 700 award winners what I had just learned.

WHAT HEALTH IS to the individual, morale is to the corporation. Health, as defined by the World Health Organization, is not merely the absence of disease or infirmity. "It is a state of complete physical, mental and social well-being."

Health is the vital principle that enables us to meet and overcome the challenges of the day. For this, medicine and surgery are not enough. Preventive measures are only part of the picture. We must enlist all our functions, bring together body, mind and spirit to attain true health. This global approach is holistic medicine. It is medicine that sees the entire life-style of the individual as important.

The same concept is now taking place in industry. Morale is no less than corporate health. It is the vital principle within a company that enables it to meet and overcome the challenges of the business day. For this, science and technology are not enough. The hard factors of production, capital investment, research and development are only part of the picture. It is necessary to enlist the soft factors—motivation, job satisfaction and collaboration —to attain true morale. This global approach could be called holistic management. It sees the entire life-style of the corporation as important.

The Japanese have become masters at this. They have the hard factors in productivity. Their mastery, however, is due to the soft factors, those concerned with the human problems in productivity. The basic quality that is needed here is trust. Then there is subtlety, an acknowledgment that each individual must be accepted as a unique complex of experiences, attitudes and prejudices. Finally, there is an intimacy, a feeling of union with the others in the plant.

The Japanese do have a culture that contains and reinforces all these qualities. We live in a quite different social setting. While the Japanese have order dictated by a regard for their tradition and ancestors, we have order prescribed by law.

The two social orders are worlds apart in their effect on morale. Morale is cooperative determination, and Japanese culture reinforces and enriches it. Law creates the opposite effect. Law creates the determination not to cooperate, not to unite, but to disagree.

The law does not heal wounds, it causes them. It does not create relationships, it destroys them. The law is a poor substitute for the peace that comes from identifying with others. We live in a country, work at plants and reside in homes where life is becoming an adversary situation. It is not I and Thou; it is I *or* Thou.

Our need is for management and labor to develop our own versions of trust and subtlety and intimacy. Technical skill and skill with people rarely go hand in hand. We need supervisors and administrators who have the right instinct for people, who are experts in those things that cannot be taught and know just what to do and say when facing another human being.

Primarily, they must care and make that caring felt. The workers must know that the corporation cares. That is the role of holistic management: great involvement with every employee in the organization. How this will be developed will differ in almost every instance, but the desire and commitment alone can be decisive.

I once had as a patient an elderly Russian lady whose apartment was a profusion of beautiful plants and flowers. On the floor above her lived a woman whose plants just would not grow. She looked for advice from my patient, who told her she must love her plants for them to flourish.

"I tell my plants, 'I love you,' " my patient said to me, "and they know I do. She tells hers, 'I love you, I love you,' but they don't grow. They know she doesn't really love them."

Love has nothing to do with logic. Caring has nothing to do with technology. Yet without love and caring there will be no health in the individual or morale in the corporation.

Chapter Fifteen
On Aging

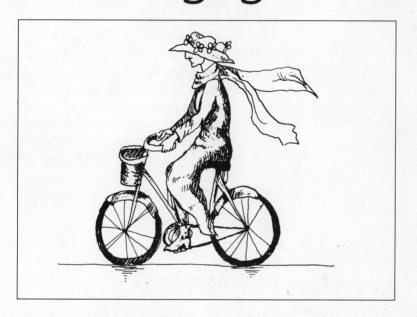

"Most people live nowhere near their limits.
They settle for an accelerated aging, an early
and precipitous fall. They give aging a bad
name. Too many people entering their
forties are performing at physiological levels
more appropriate to somebody sixty years
old."

WHEN I TOOK UP RUNNING at the age of forty-five I joined a high school cross-country team. I had to. There were no older runners in my area and extremely few competitive events. So I kept my gear in my car and would consult the local paper for the time and place of the high school meets.

My teammates quickly accepted me. At the races it was a different story. The opposing teams and their coaches would find it quite odd that someone my age would be running and actually competing. In the races, I invariably had to pass a runner twice. The first time he would be startled and immediately spurt ahead. The second time I would put him away.

These young runners had not yet had their consciousness raised to the marvelous capability of the human body. Nor, indeed, had anyone else. In those days older runners were eccentrics, especially in cross-country season, when they might appear in longjohns on the roads. No one, including these aging runners, had any idea how little attrition occurs to the human machine with aging.

Those young athletes I ran with had a sense of urgency about their performances which I did not have. They would talk to me about two more years or one more year of eligibility. They saw their participation limited to the scholastic career; meanwhile my body was telling me to take the long view. This running, it said, can go on forever. It was that body wisdom that dispelled my preconceptions about aging. Just as women later took to running despite centuries of pronouncements to the contrary. And when they did I took the role of my high school doubters. Now it was me that a woman had to pass twice. And just as the younger runners finally grasped the truth, so did I. Women of all ages not only can run, they run well. Some of them run exceptionally well.

Now races are filled with runners over forty years of age of both sexes. The average times turned in by these older athletes are remarkable. They demonstrate just how gradual is the loss of running ability as age progresses. The study on master runners conducted by Washington University School of Medicine in St. Louis, in which I am a subject, has shown the decline to be only about 5 percent a decade.

What does this all mean? It depends upon your age. If you are a high school runner, you can see that your athletic career need never end. Indeed it must not. In physiology you get what you pay for. The effects of aging are minor as long as you keep your training and weight constant. You can be an athlete at any age, but you have to work at it.

Those who are older and have deserted exercise and play and sport must get back to it. This is the time to spend your unspent youth. There is no physiological reason to accept the rocking chair and the slippers. The minimal changes due to age would not be apparent in the course of the normal active day.

Fortunately this training need take little time. The fitness requirement is half an hour of movement at a comfortable pace four times a week. The master runners do more than that, of course, and their movement is running. But even for them the outlay is little more than four hours a week devoted to this training.

Such activity is needed to satisfy the animal in us. It is what is necessary to make you and me good animals. And that forms the base from which we can operate. Given a sound and healthy and fit body, we can pursue perfection in various ways. Once we have acquired the energy to make the day easy and the crisis conquerable, age will become the youth we were promised when we were young.

WHEN I BEGAN RUNNING I became my own coach. I had to. At that time, no one was interested in the training of a middle-aged runner. No one was writing about the conditioning of older athletes.

It was left to me to decide on goals and a training schedule. I had to determine the correct frequency and intensity and duration of my workouts. I was an experiment of one. And lacking both instruction and experience, I was forced to learn through my mistakes.

There is a saying in medical school that if you treat yourself, you have a fool for a patient. The same thing applies to coaching.

Someone has to keep his head while you are losing yours. Someone must resist the pressure of pride and ambition, of wishful thinking and dreams of glory. Someone must stand back and see things as they are. Someone must make the difficult decisions. It takes a sound mind to train a sound body. And when ego is involved, sanity is likely to go out the window.

I was no different from many others. I immediately fell into the pit. I committed all the cardinal sins of coaching.

My first and most serious transgression was to set unreasonable goals. I was influenced in this by my early success. There is always that initial quantum jump in running ability. The ease with which I progressed from a brisk walk to an easy two miles persuaded me that such improvement would follow an upward line to infinity.

Once I was running well, I expected to run better and better: break five minutes in the mile; go under three hours in the marathon; catch up to those youngsters twenty-five years my junior. I looked for too much, too soon.

Unreasonable goals mean unreasonable training. I had hardly broken in my shoes when I was caught in the mileage trap. I was soon putting in more weekly distance than I had done on a championship cross-country team in college. When not doing distance on the road, I did interval work on the track and then ranged anywhere within a two-hour drive of my home looking for weekly road races.

The inevitable occurred again and again: recurrent staleness, exhaustion, sickness. I finally realized that the more I did, the worse I became. I discovered that Selye was right. The body can be trained to greater performance through application of stress. But the amount of stress and the time allowed for recovery are critical to the success of this process.

Being self-coached, I developed injuries. Again, these come as part of high goals and heavy training schedules. Long mileage, hills and speedwork breed injuries. I went through shin splints and Achilles tendinitis, runner's knee and the heel-spur syndrome. Worse, I tended to ignore them. Like many another runner, I ran hurt. I would not let an injury or an illness make me miss a race for which I had trained for months.

This attitude is almost universal. The glamor events in road running always have their share of runners who would be better off as spectators. They compete despite an illness or an injury or total exhaustion. I had a telephone call from just such a runner in South Africa two days before the 56-mile Comrade's Marathon. He had gone through a week-long fever of such severity that the doctors had seen fit to do a spinal tap to rule out encephalitis. "Would it be all right," he asked, "to run the Comrade's?" He had been in training for this race for six months and could not bear to miss it.

When he finished his question, I asked one in return. "Do you have a family?" Only someone alone in this world, whose survival mattered only to himself, would run the Comrade's in that condition.

It is quite difficult when you are your own coach to take the long view, to understand that running is a lifetime activity. Short-term triumphs matter very little. There will always be another race, another marathon, another Comrade's, even another Boston. It is possible to miss the race next Sunday and survive.

I eventually lowered my goals. I know now that athletes are much like racing cars and racing boats. We have a built-in range of performance. There is, it is true, a continuing slow improvement over the years. But year in and year out, I see the same bodies around me as I near the end of a race.

Eventually I also modified my training, just as I had modified my goals. I took one day off a week, then two. Now I do as little as 30 miles a week and find I can still race well, even continue to improve. I limit my intervals to those few weeks before the three or four races a year that I want to run especially well. The times when I run well don't spur me to train more. Nor does a bad performance get me out early the next day to put in extra miles.

However, if I made mistakes, there were compensations. In time, I came to see the other values in running. Being my own coach taught me to be independent, to trust my own experience, to learn from my own mistakes. Being a coach made me an expert on myself.

The mistakes I made in coaching were no worse than the mis-

takes I had made in living: unreasonable goals, misguided efforts, the short-term view, the failure to recognize what is
important. I see that now. Running not only made me a coach; it
made me a philosopher.

WHEN A FRIEND OF MINE, a former Olympic skier, passed the
landmark age of thirty, she took herself off chronological time.
Now, if asked how old she is, she answers, "My biological age is
nineteen."

It is the biological or, better, the *physiological* age that matters. Despite the passage of years, the body can stay young
functionally. If a person continues to train for maximum performance, a smooth trajectory can be plotted: a rising curve from
adolescence to a peak at about the age of twenty-eight and then
a slow decline to the biblical age and beyond.

Most people live nowhere near their limits. They settle for an
accelerated aging, an early and precipitous fall. They give aging
a bad name. Too many people entering their forties are performing at physiological levels more appropriate to somebody sixty
years old.

It is time to elevate our consciousness of normal aging. Normal
is the best you can be at any age. The normal forty-year-old is
capable of athletic performances within 95 percent of the healthy
twenty-five-year-old. The age group record for the marathon is
within 95 percent of the world record.

And this relationship holds as the years go on. The group
running records at age fifty are 85 percent of the world's records.
Those at sixty are 75 percent. And one should realize that millions are attempting to set world records. A relative handful are
competing at the age group levels.

These record holders are, I will grant, motor geniuses. Nevertheless, the same principle holds for us lesser folk. Whatever our
personal world record might have been at the age of twenty-five,
we can now approach it in our forties and fifties and sixties and
even seventies to the same extent that these superathletes do.
We can come within 5 or 15 or 25 percent of our peak performance.

I know this to be true from my own experience. I was a 4:20 miler in college. A secondary runner who filled in on the two-mile relay; no great shakes. Yet when I train down fine I can equal the statistics I have just presented to you. I have over the years shown the gradual reduction in performance that would be anticipated. At fifty I ran a 4:47 mile. At sixty, the equivalent of a 5:10.

I am now part of a study designed to document these changes through laboratory tests. Dr. John Holloszy and his associates at the Washington University School of Medicine in St. Louis have recruited a group of 16 master runners, averaging fifty-nine years of age, and matched us with 16 young athletes having much the same ability we had in our college days. I am, for instance, teamed up with a twenty-two-year-old, a 4.22 miler.

Each group has gone through a battery of tests. Maximum oxygen uptakes, percentage body-fat determinations, and echo-cardiograms were done to establish our current levels of fitness. When my results were compared to those of my younger alter ego, the investigators discovered that I had deteriorated about 5 percent a decade from my peak. And this proved to be the average lowering of function for each of the master runners.

This study has been an eye opener to the physiologists. The generally accepted figure for physiological aging is about 9 percent a decade. Some reports show even greater losses. Years ago, Sidney Robinson, an outstanding worker in the field of exercise physiology, studied the effects of age on a number of nationally ranked runners. At the average age of forty-eight they had lost up to forty-two percent of the capability that had brought them to prominence.

Robinson published his findings under the title "The Physiological Aging of Champion Runners." In retrospect, we can see the source of his error. These figures were not attributable to the normal physiological effects of aging. They were the abnormal effects. These world-class runners were heavy smokers. Their natural talent had succumbed to sedentary living. They were not aging. They were rusting out. Some were rotting out.

Only when training and weight and health states are constant can the actual effects of aging be charted. The research done at

St. Louis puts normal physiological aging at just about 5 percent per decade. It confirms what my running had already told me. You can use your own body to make sure that your physiological and chronological age coincide.

I am simply a normal sixty-three-year-old getting the physiological limit out of my body. My biological age is sixty-three. My friend, the ex-Olympian, has a biological age of thirty, not nineteen. She has the capabilities of her thirty-year-old body trained to its peak.

Being an Olympian may make a difference. Not in ability, which is, in any case, relative, but in attitude. When you are thinking: higher, faster, farther, you seldom worry whether some things may be out of your reach.

When people suggest you act your age, you do . . . and go for it.

"No WISE MAN," I said, quoting Jonathan Swift, "ever wished to be younger." The 300 or so runners in my audience nodded their wise heads in agreement. It was one of those speeches I frequently give to runners the night before a race. What was different was these runners. They were, all of them, men and women over forty years of age. The race the next day was a 5-kilometer event limited to this age group: Master runners.

I stood there looking out at those bright young faces. These were people who had found what age had to offer and found it good, who had discovered that age always contains what has gone before. The sixties, said one sage, contain the twenties and the forties. Proust put it more poetically: "Man is a creature without any fixed age who has the faculty of becoming in a few seconds many years younger." We can each of us at any moment relive anything that happened to us during our life span.

We Masters, I told them, have acquired a repertoire of qualities and capabilities the young cannot match. Age is constantly conferring new privileges, new abilities, new insights. We have grown in wisdom and experience. We are now superior to the individuals we were in our youth. And yet we have sacrificed very little. Only in a physical sense are we inferior to those people we were in our twenties. And even there, as tomorrow would show, few in that age group can equal our deeds. Most runners in the room tonight were in better physical condition than at any previous time in their lives.

My sixties did indeed include my twenties. Tomorrow I would be twenty again. In running that race I would relive races I had run in college. I would feel the same excitement, the same surge of adrenalin, the same challenges, the same pain, the same exhaustion, the same terrible shortness of breath, the same heaviness in the legs. The same exquisite satisfaction and relief in finally crossing the line.

My sixties also include my thirties. I remember what it was like not to be a runner, not to be an athlete. I remember those dormant days doing the work of the hive, waiting, although I did not know it, for the fullness that would come with the return to play and sport. Feeling all the while the death of ambition and the dissatisfaction with success.

Those listening to me knew my talk before I gave it. They had lived it just as I had. They knew the advantage they had over the young. We could be young, but they could not be old. They cannot know what we now know, cannot have the certainty we have acquired through the years of uncertainty.

What we lose with age, said Emerson, we can afford to lose. In our passage through the years we have focused on what is important. We have discarded the second rate. We have learned that trivia is indeed trivia. We have dispensed with tricks. We have not aged as much as we have moved from one age to another. The French speak of a third age. There is the age of the student. The age of the worker. And this third age of those ready to enjoy the fruits of study and work. The Masters.

We are indeed Masters, I told them. We are professors. We are professionals. We have come into maturity. And we have matured doing what appears to be childish things. Nevertheless, our ability to live with questions and without solutions began when we took to the roads. Our belief in ourselves and in living our own lives developed through our running. It was running that released the treasures in our subconscious and gave us the creativity to put these treasures in substantial form.

Keep running, I told the forties and fifties and sixties looking up at me, the best is indeed yet to come.

PERHAPS BEING OVER SIXTY years of age makes me more sensitive, but no matter how people praise old age I notice a touch of condescension. They give me the feeling of someone watching another human being in difficulty and marveling at how well he is handling it. Age is never considered a gift. It is one of those natural disasters that must be met, and, if possible, with equanimity. No one seems to understand that age is the ultimate peak experience. It is the time of life for which all else is preparation.

The failure to appreciate the superiority of old age is due in part to the identification of age with death. Yet as we can see from the daily obituary columns, death comes at any time. Only a few are prepared for it. The artist, the athlete, the saint and the aged. They share a common experience. They know that after the absolutely superb effort, after a personal best, after the peak experience, comes physical and creative and spiritual exhaustion. There is a morning-after when all is ashes. It is not worth the effort to get out of bed. The hero of the day before has become an ant.

These deaths to the self and our ambitions, these periods of mourning for our hopes and our desires, come along regularly. No age is free of them. Only the elders have come to expect and welcome them. In such days are the seeds of new beginnings. They are invariably followed by new insights, new ideas, new concepts, new achievements. The progress of man is cyclical, and the peaks of that progress, not death, occupy the aging.

The major exponents of this attitude toward aging are the "young-old" described by psychiatrist Bernice Naughton. "The young-old," she writes, "are a rapidly growing group of retirees and their spouses who are physically and mentally vigorous and whose major characteristic is a new leisure time. They are people seeking interesting ways to use their time, both for self-fulfillment and for contributing to their communities."

The young-old constitutes a new aristocracy, a new leisure class pursuing truth. Their leisure is in the Greek tradition: time given over to education, to making one's life a work of art. It is an evocation, a heightening of the qualities that one implicitly possesses.

We aging see the environment as one that rewards boldness and risk taking. We bring to bear in any situation the gifts and the emotions, the strengths and the enthusiasm, of any of the ages we have gone through. We can now play any role. We have played them all before.

This is not to imply that we know it all. But it is to say we have lost nothing and we have gained freedoms we never anticipated. Further, we are no longer faceless youths barely distinguishable one from the other. Each of us is an original. Our bodies and minds and spirits are the unique expression of a personality in the final stages of evolution.

I said I could play any role. What is necessary is the script. When I was young I used other playwrights. I accepted the play and the role assigned to me. Now it is different. This is my play. This is my script. This is no role; this is me. The years in rehearsal, the decades in preparation, all the hard work, all those mistakes, are now paying off.

Now you know our secret. No young-old wants to be young again. We just want to feel young.

Chapter Sixteen
On Choosing

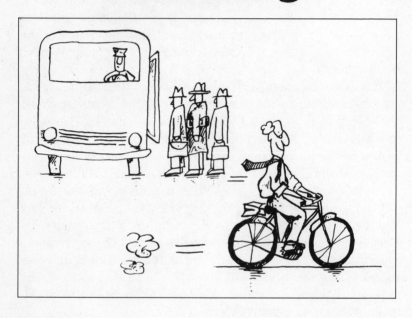

"Your body reveals you within and without. It tells the perceptive observer your philosophy, your view of the universe."

WHEN I TALK to college students, I preach heresy. I use heresy in the sense of the original Greek, which means choice. I preach their abiding, permanent and absolute need for choice.

Some of that never-ending responsibility they already recognize. Other preachers have spoken of the obligation to choose from the alternatives of good and evil, industry and sloth. The sermons of our youth were filled with the should's and ought's of law and duty and culture.

That is not choice but acceptance. It is not adding to our life. It limits it. Our obedience to the rule, our acceptance of the regulation maintains our traditions, our institutions, our society. It furthers identity. It reduces individuality.

The heresy I present to them begins with the body. In our present academy the body is ignored. Physical education, basic to the education of aristocrats whether they lived in Athens in the fifth century B.C. or Florence during the Renaissance or Boston at the turn of the century, is no longer important.

When George Leonard, writer on human potential, visits college campuses he usually asks to meet with the physical educators. His faculty hosts are amazed. What in the world is to be gained by that? They regard attention to the body and play and sports as diversions from the real task of the university.

I ask these students to reexamine that idea and choose the body. Not to the exclusion of the mind and soul but in conjunction with them. To see themselves as evolving wholes. Body and mind expressing the personality that is the self.

The aristocrats in Greece embraced that unity. "Arete," the root of the word "aristocrat," means to fulfill one's function, to become whatever you are. We are wholes. Body, mind and soul.

The body cannot be ignored. The body is me, I am my body. The portrait painter Alice Neale tells us how much can be seen in a face. "I paint the inside as well as the outside. I paint the person's philosophy." Your body reveals you within and without. It tells the perceptive observer your philosophy, your view of the universe.

My body can expand my life or diminish it. To live totally I must be an athlete. I must follow the laws that govern the body. When I opt for the body, I accept the obligation of training it.

Higher education, I suggest, should consist of training both mind and body, one quite as rigorously as the other. William James, one of the great American thinkers, firmly believed in this. "I hope that the ideal of the well-trained and vigorous body," said James, "will be maintained neck and neck with that of the well-trained and vigorous mind as two co-equal halves in the higher education for men and women."

The psychological and philosophical reasons for a well-trained body were deeply important to James. Yet the physiological reasons are, at least initially, greater.

"The body," as Plato said, "is the source of all energy and initiative." The trained body gives us the maximum available energy, provides us with the most powerful initiative. Why place ourselves at a disadvantage? Are we going to get the most out of the person we are—or aren't we?

In his talk on "The Energies of Man" James speaks of our defection. In perhaps the most telling phrase in all his work he said, "We lead lives inferior to ourselves." Not, I tell the students, inferior to the leading scholar or the leading activist or the leading artist or even the leading athletes in this institution. Not to the number-one person in any of those fields—but to the self each one of us can and should be.

Abraham Maslow once suggested that we study the "good choosers." Those "gold medalists" who make work a pleasure, duty a delight, and turn selfishness into altruism. That is the definition, it seeems to me, of a good and healthy narcissism. Choose well, I urge the heretics-to-be in front of me. Choose yourself, but choose your body first. Become an athlete, the person James called "a secular saint."

IN 1898, WILLIAM JAMES stated that our physical breakdowns were due to the turbulence of our inner environment. In 1961, Dr. Meyer Friedman agreed with him. He reported a correlation between type-A behavior and coronary artery heart disease.

Type-A people, Friedman said, are engaged in a chronic incessant endeavor to accomplish more and more in less and less time. This "hurry sickness" was usually associated with a free-floating hostility ready to vent itself at the slightest provocation.

This behavior apparently has widespread multiple adverse metabolic effects. These are generally known as coronary risk factors, and most of us are familiar with them. Elevation of cholesterol, triglycerides and adrenalin substances are perhaps the best known. The probability is that even more will be detected in the future.

The medical reaction has been to attack the branches, not the roots. Steps are taken in hopes of lowering cholesterol. Efforts are made to reduce hypertension. Type-A people are encouraged to stop smoking. As each leak occurs in the dike, there is a concerted move to plug it up.

Such measures appear to Friedman to be absurd. "Attempts are being made to prevent initial or recurrent coronary heart disease by ignoring its chief cause," he writes. Physicians, he says, are concentrating solely on secondary biophysical and biomechanical abnormalities or the noxious habit patterns possibly generated by this same overlooked cause. The solution is to modify type-A behavior and thus reduce the coronary risk.

James was in full agreement with this position. In his Gospel of Relaxation he spoke again and again of changing our inner climate. He spoke out for training the body and championed a physical training equal to that of the mind. His cure for hurry sickness was to become physically fit.

Stating what should be done is not the same as doing it. Lowering cholesterol is child's play to modifying behavior. James was preaching to the converted, graduating class of the Boston School of Gymnastics. Friedman says his best results are with people who have already suffered a heart attack. Nobody wants to be saved until salvation appears lost.

Until a person has a heart attack the very idea of having one appears inconceivable. Indeed, the first reaction the heart-attack victim has is disbelief. "This cannot possibly be a heart attack," one says to oneself. All manner of ills are considered. I know of physicians who explained away their pain and went back to chopping wood, or ate a sumptuous meal, or claimed it was all due to bursitis.

The difficulty of the problem should not dissuade us from the conclusion reached by both James and Friedman. If you wish to reduce all risk you must change behavior. It's our attitude that raises the cholesterol. Our emotions that elevate the blood pressure. Our inner storms that lead us to cigarettes.

For Friedman this change is a matter of spending time with the patient, convincing the potential victim that this life-style is self-defeating. James would have us find this out for ourselves. Use the body, train it, perfect it, and you will find your behavior changing with that perfection.

Many teachers would agree with James, the teacher. They know that nothing worth learning can be taught. They realize that anything that changes behavior must be self-experienced. Do not argue. Do not debate. Simply motivate. Induce them to experience their bodies, become fit, learn how to play, engage in sport. Your work will be done.

Friedman would redeem his patients through convincing them of the error of their ways. Most type-A people, he discovered, are proud of their hurry sickness and attribute their success to this dedication to work. Friedman would show them otherwise. Type-A behavior does not bring success and it breeds emotional and spiritual disease.

His tack is to convince type-A people of two things: that their success, whatever it is, is due to their other attributes—creativity, organization, professional skill. The hurry sickness has nothing to do with it. And, secondly, that this incessant single-focused pursuit has limited their growth in other areas. They are emotionally and creatively deprived. Friedman states it more plainly. They have, he says, a spiritual illness.

Reading James, I get the same impression. Here is human potential going down the drain. And neither of these men will have it. But being on the side of the angels is not enough. Good intentions are not enough. How can a life be changed?

Not by words. At least that is my belief. Or if by words, they are the perfect words to express what you have already experienced. In this Friedman may succeed. He may, by his words, recall to the person what it was like in the past. He will bring up the conversion-creating experience.

James suggests we create the experience and the desired conversion will follow. Exercise the body, train the muscles, and in due time we will find a mental health to go along with the physical one.

James telescopes this process. He suggests it is as simple as Friedman admits it is difficult. It is not all that simple. It occurs in stages. Each of them must be lived through and then the next step is taken. But millions of people have tried it and have been successful. Everyday I meet people who have gone back to their bodies and found the self they were meant to be.

CHOICE ALWAYS LEADS to more choice. The heretics who opt for training the body discover that other doors must be opened. The first leads to play. Training, they find, is enough for the body. It does give energy and vitality. There is a new presence. One becomes a good animal. Training becomes a means to this end.

The choice now comes in the expression of this evolving personality. The traditional view of normality is the ability to love and to work. From Freud and his theories to George Valiant's studies of Harvard graduates, the ability to love and to work remains the chief criterion in measuring adaptation to various life situations. The graduates with stable marriages and job satisfaction had the best mental health.

There is, however, a third choice, again complementary to the other two, which is play. Play provides the third dimension—creativity. In the playful use of our bodies, we give release to the treasures in our subconscious, the experiences stored there since birth. "Genius," said James, "is simply a different way of looking at things." It is a genius we all possess and can make available in play.

In all too many instances we fear we have no inherent creativity. Yet this is not true. "If most of us tend to keep on going [through] the same familiar motions, this is not because we are short on creativity, but because we stifle it." So wrote the late Lawrence Kubie. In commenting on this observation, Bill Moyers suggests: "Discover the impediment, exorcise it, and creativity will flow."

The impediments are many, but a playful, well-trained body removes most of them. There is a special case to be made for motion. "Never trust a thought you came upon sitting down," said Nietzsche. "The muscles must be in celebration with the mind." Thoreau made a similar statement: "It seems when my legs begin walking, my mind begins working . . . any writing I do sitting down is wooden." The play of the body, as surely as purposeless walking is play, leads to the play of the mind we call creativity.

The education that stifles play stifles creativity. Play therefore becomes what Peter Berger calls a heretical imperative. We may refuse to train our bodies or subsequently use them in play, but we should be aware of the choice and all its implications. There should be informed consent.

Most consent is uninformed. Why else this endless flow from lecture to lecture, followed by long hours of study—and only a trickle to the gymnasium and the playing fields. The Greeks knew better. An hour a day at the gymnasium or palestra was the rule. Some of the Roman intellectuals like Seneca had their own trainers.

Nietzsche, who believed in motion, also believed in play. "All great ideas are conceived in play." Man's most important activity, said Hoffer. The primary energy of man, said Ortega, was sportive or playful.

Moyers, in studying creativity, describes the attributes leading to this quality. Creative people, he discovered, tolerate ambiguity, are willing to take risks, have a strong sense of self, a need to prove their worth and, finally, discipline.

A quick perusal of these attributes should make it clear that they are common also to those individuals who have trained their bodies and discovered their play. They are the basic characteristics of the "good choosers" described by Maslow.

Ultimately, however, training and play will be insufficient. Creativity is not simply concerned with novelty. What comes from seeing the old as new must be a transforming development, an evolution or unfolding of the self. For that to happen we must make another choice: risk.

Risk is a moral equivalent to war. James and others, notably Ernest Becker, have seen clearly our need to be heroes. We require, therefore, an arena for heroism, a theater where we can act out our drama as the person we want to be.

That arena is sport. Athletics are the moral equivalent of war, our games the theater for heroism. George Santayana, that urbane Harvard philosopher and most unlikely supporter of such ideas, spoke strongly to this view in his "Philosophy on the Bleachers."

"It is not the mere need of healthy exercise that brings the players," said Santayana. "Athletics have a higher function than gymnastics and deeper basis than utility." Santayana saw the intimate relation between games and war, but he observed that "the games arose from the comparative freedom from war, and the consequent liberation of martial energy from the stimulus of necessity, and the expression of it in beautiful and spectacular forms."

The martial virtues are what we need when we place ourselves at risk. To do what will be beautiful and spectacular we must be "Spartan, active, courageous, capable of serious enthusiasm and ready to endure discipline."

In Cambridge in 1894, Santayana saw sports as the student's salvation. "Our athletic life," he stated, "is the most conspicuous and promising rebellion against this industrial tyranny"—the conformity in the United States. Now, almost a century later, it is the most promising rebellion against academic tyranny.

If we are to be heroes, and heroes we must be, sports offer us the preeminent arena in which to achieve this status. As we have so often been told, it is not in winning or losing we become heroes but in the way we play the game. The risk is always there. But the risk is not in losing to an opponent: it is in losing to your lesser self.

Oddly, this rarely happens. Just as in war there are cowards but little cowardice, so in sports there are quitters who refuse to quit. In sports the heroic becomes the commonplace.

Once we have experienced the heroic we are never the same, that experience enters our subconscious, becomes part of our memory both verbal and nonverbal (or mystical). The heroic experience becomes both source and reason for our creativity.

It is the hero who tolerates ambiguity, who is willing to take risks. The hero has a strong sense of self, a need to prove his worth and discipline. It is the hero who has all the attributes of the creative person.

Part Two
The
ATHLETIC
EXPERIENCE

Chapter Seventeen
On Meaning

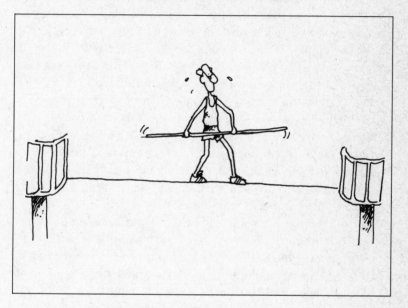

"We need all three activities. Exercise is a science. Play is an art. Sport is both. Exercise is mechanical. Play is free-flowing. Sport is exercise with rules and a reckoning at the finish. Sport is exercise with consequences."

WHEN I LECTURE on fitness I admit up front that running is boring. I know that a majority of the people in the audience hold that opinion. Many have come to that conclusion simply by observing joggers on the road. Others have actually tried running and found it to be drudgery. I am usually facing a group of people who either failed in fitness programs or never got started.

The major obstacle to a successful fitness program is boredom, the feeling of wanting to be doing something else. When you are bored you are acutely aware there are much more interesting or satisfying things to do. Places, people and activities bore you because at this very minute you want to be elsewhere. An elsewhere with pleasure and excitement and absorption. An elsewhere without feelings of inadequacy and embarrassment and discomfort. An elsewhere where you feel at home.

My object is to suggest to the people in the audience how they can be made to feel at home in a fitness program. That program, if it is to succeed, must be interesting and satisfying. It should be filled with pleasure and excitement and absorption. It must be a place where a person is rarely if ever bored.

Can all this be accomplished while doing something boring? Possibly. You might, for instance, try thinking of something interesting while you are doing something boring. If the running movement can be made automatic, the mind then can wander through meadows of thought, completely engrossed in its own activities. This is called dissociation, and most runners do it. When you see them trotting down the road, their minds are usually miles and possibly centuries away.

I find swimming boring because I am unable to dissociate while I swim. The instant I let my mind go off on its own, I sink. I have to attend constantly to the movement of my arms and legs or I flounder in the water. When I run, however, I am able to put my body on automatic pilot and let my mind loose to search for interesting ideas.

If this fails you can try another ploy. Make what is boring interesting. Take an interesting companion on the run. Good talk can halve the distance. You will come to the end of the run feeling as if you had just begun. If you are a gossip you should run with a gossip. If people form a large part of your world, your fitness world must include them as well.

Another way to make something boring interesting is to make it competitive. In running, for instance, you can add the race. An entry blank can introduce you to a new and intensely absorbing world. The jogging during the week then has a new spur, a new motive—performance against your peers.

There are races and there is The Race—the marathon. Many runners who would have been dropouts have stayed in the sport because of this 26.2 mile challenge . . . the Everest of distance running. The marathon raises running out of the ordinary and commonplace and puts it in the Olympic category. Running becomes an epic event, a place for heroes.

In many instances these measures fail; people still do not want to run. Covert Bailey, the author of *Fit or Fat* and a great proponent of running, tells of a friend's coming up to him and saying, "Covert, there is no getting away from it, running is boring."

"No, John," said Covert, "you're boring. You are so boring you can't spend a half hour alone with yourself."

Nevertheless, the truth is that there are no boring people. Those we consider bores are simply interested in subjects that are of no interest to us. In a fitness program this means searching for something interesting to do. If running cannot be made interesting, then perhaps cycling or swimming or cross country skiing can be. There are people who were repeated dropouts in a variety of activities until they discovered karate or weight lifting or aerobic dancing. Or racquet ball.

When pushed into a corner, I ask the audience to remember what they enjoyed doing as children. That form of play or something similar to it will still be satisfying to the body. If you then add the socialization or competition that you need, fitness will come without any further concern on your part. And you will seldom be bored in the process.

AT BIRTH we are all generalists. As children we are curious about everything. We insist on exploring and exploiting all our abilities. We run and play, we sing and dance, we write and draw without thought as to whether or not we are good at it. Our games change with the seasons. Our lives are lived in a classroom that is the world. This allows for an infinite variety of physical expression.

As time passes we become specialists. We constrict our interests, narrow our participation. We limit the expression of the self. This happens in our mental life. It happens in our creative life. It happens in our physical life. We find one occupation, one avocation, one sport. Everything else that is human becomes foreign to us.

This is the major indictment of distance runners. Not that we are narcissistic, but that we are so obsessed with running we devote no time to the rest of our body. We do not develop its varied strengths and skills. We never learn the other ways the body can speak and experience, can teach and be taught.

We are not alone. Most present-day athletes are specialists. They concentrate on their sport as we do on running. They, too, congregate together, speaking in their own tongue, demanding allegiance. They also are sects who see others as heathens or heretics or backsliders lost forever to the truth.

Runners do not understand why everyone is not a runner. Cyclists feel the same way about cycling. Golfers about golf. Tennis players about tennis. Each sport has its passionate advocates who have found the Grail and see no reason why they should try anything else.

Were we the children we were meant to be, we would enjoy all sports. Were we the generalists that we once were, we would delight in all the things the body loves to do. We would play the games that have withstood the test of time and progress.

I am now incapable of sports in which I was once proficient. Up until now I did not care. Running was enough. Now I am not so sure. In putting on the New Man, must I not also develop all the things the body can do? and should I not rejoin all those friends I dismissed on my way to becoming a distance runner? Is not the glory of God man who is really functioning—not merely running?

The prominence given the decathlon is one answer to these questions. The winner of the decathlon is the hero of each Olympiad. He is the athlete we remember. Yet the decathlete is a person who is fairly good at everything and rarely exceptional at anything. The decathlete is mediocrity lived and at its highest standard. The decathlete is the generalist raised to the highest level. The decathlete is the best common man.

We common men will find no better inspiration. We are better at some sports than others, but we are not really hotshots at anything. Instead of concentrating on one area of mediocrity we should vary our sports and enlarge our physical experience. We will come to know our bodies in new and satisfying mediocre ways.

The number of athletes, young and old, participating in multiple sports is growing. That is as it should be. Athletes, not poets, are the antenna of the race. The body teaches more clearly than any other agent. In childhood that meant total sports activity. Adults unfortunately take longer to learn. We have to go through being specialists before we become the generalists and decathletes we once were.

THE SPORTS PSYCHOLOGISTS had invited me to Ottawa to present an address at their international meeting. For the first time in their history, a section was being devoted to the personal meaning of sports through life. The rest of the meeting, as always, would focus on ways to enhance athletic development.

Sports psychologists can presently be classified into two distinct groups: those doing scientific studies and experimental work in sports, and those who deliver the clinical service before, during and after competition. Both groups concentrate on athletes and their problems. Both operate in a framework which deals exclusively with the athlete's performance.

My thesis was that the psychologists had taken a parochial view of their specialty. They did not recognize the full scope of their discipline, either in the range of people it should treat or in the type of activities it should cover. Two things could remedy this:

One was to consider every person a potential athlete. Thus the influence of the psychologist would extend to everyone who could have his consciousness raised to his athletic and human potential.

The other was for psychologists to extend their sports practice to include both exercise and play. These three distinct but inter-related activities would have to be understood and then inte-grated if sports psychology were to have a beneficial effect on the present fitness craze.

We know all the physiology we need to know to become fit. We know next to nothing, however, about the *psychology* of fitness. When we regiment people, it is easy to get them fit. What we can't do is induce them to do it on their own. We haven't devised the psychological supports needed to make fitness pro-grams successful.

Our difficulty is not in performance but in motivation, not in world records or personal bests, but in the desire and the disci-pline to stay with the training required to lead the athletic life. We need expert psychological help to increase participation and then prevent dropping out.

I am not a scientist, I told these scientists. I am a specimen. I am an example of what happens when a person finds his sport and persists in it. The last twenty years have been a learning, growing period of my life. It has been marked by an awareness of what is possible for me. I have discovered new levels of per-formance and new feelings about myself and my body. And I have been able to express this experience in new and creative ways.

I have done this by rediscovering the athlete I was in my youth. But this time I learned from my body. I listened to what was going on inside me. I saw the effect that my running was having, not only on my body-brain complex, but also on the self that this body and brain expressed.

I learned something I always knew but did not remember: the difference between exercise and play and sports. Each is a separate and distinct entity, each with its own function, each essential and fundamental to our nature. Each fulfills in some way our need to demonstrate who we are. Each makes us feel better about ourselves and the life we lead.

For too long people have tended to use the words interchangeably.

"Does anyone here," I asked the psychologists, "know how to play this game? Does anyone here understand the difference between exercise, play and sport?"

Do you, my reader?

OF THE THREE athletic activities—exercise, play and sport— exercise is the easiest to define. Exercise is work. In the words of Mark Twain, it is anything a body does not want to do. Exercise is dull and boring and an extremely slow way to pass the time. Exercise is counting repetitions and watching the clock. Exercise is waiting until it ends.

We all understand exercise. It is the phys. ed. we were given in school. It is the fitness programs offered us today. Exercise is pure physiology with nothing to make it palatable. Exercising consistently, therefore, requires some of the martial virtues: discipline, a sense of obligation, a realization that the results will make boredom and fatigue and suffering worthwhile. Exercise has purpose, but it has no meaning.

Play and sports are the opposite. They have meaning but no purpose. From there on, however, they differ. And that difference, unfortunately, is not generally recognized. We often use the words "play" and "sport" synonymously. There is no verb for "sport." So we use the word "play" in attempting to describe sport. We say we *play* tennis. Or we say we *play* football. But we're not playing at all. When there are rules, when there is a score, when something is at risk, it is not play. It is sport.

Not to see this difference is to put yourself in one of two opposite and equally defeating situations. One is to concentrate on sports so much that play becomes nonexistent. The other is to focus on play and remove sport from your life. In either instance, you will be deprived of something essential to your development and fulfillment as a human being.

We need all three activities. Exercise is a science. Play is an art. Sport is both. Exercise is mechanical. Play is free-flowing. Sport is exercise with rules and a reckoning at the finish. Sport is exercise with consequences.

The physiologist concerned with perfecting the body and assuring maximal health need not go beyond exercise. But the fact is that few people will exercise for any length of time without the additional motive of play or sport. Most need the values introduced by play and sport to make all the training worthwhile. Then what was previously a duty becomes a privilege.

This progression can easily be seen in the runner. Running begins with fitness, 30 minutes at a comfortable pace four times a week. This makes one a jogger who exercises for no other reason than the physical benefits that come with this two hours a week. The realities of weight loss and increased energy, and the promises of longevity and freedom from heart attacks, are what motivates this beginner.

Then the jogger becomes a runner. The minutes on the run become time for meditation and creativity. City streets or rural roads become havens from the press of life and the events that promote the "hurry sickness." The daily run is no longer work, it is play.

The runner now is interested in bigger things than a low cholesterol count or normal blood pressure. The inner and outer worlds have become the focus. Running has become a search for meaning, the runs fascinating meanderings in the interstices of the mind. The sights and sounds and touches of an entire life, the subconscious ready to harvest, make every run a treasure and a delight.

But finally, even that is not enough. This search for meaning needs more. It needs a challenge, a test, an experience of the self in extremity. It needs, as William James said, a theater for heroism, a moral equivalent of war. And so the runner runs from play to sport. The runner becomes a racer.

THE DISTINCTION between play and sport may appear trivial. It is all-important. We need both. Neither alone can satisfy our inborn need for the other. There are, to be sure, certain common characteristics. Nevertheless, play and sport are different. What I ask from my body in sport becomes the source of what I create in play. Play is truly emotion recollected in tranquility. It is the art and poetry, the painting and writing—indeed any creative act—that follow from the moments when we have put ourselves at risk.

The race is sport. The race is run in a bounded area, another world operating under its own rules. And most important, the race has a closure. There are results. I am given my time and place. So the race is a perfect way to live out the trials and tests and challenges we must meet to feel good about ourselves.

There are some who would turn sport into play. Take the net down in tennis. Do not keep score in basketball. Forget about times in races. But this approach won't work. It would be disastrous to remove competition and consequences from our lives. We need them to mold us and shape us and teach us who we are and what we can become.

Sport makes us fully functioning adults. Through pushing to our limits, we grow in self-esteem and self-respect. Through doing what we do best, we attain maturity.

Play, on the other hand, returns us to childhood. It allows complete freedom. Play is unstructured and without rules. It liberates us from necessity. It asks no product, no particular performance. It refuses to be serious. Play opens up our inner world and allows our subconscious to percolate through to understanding.

For me, the race is the epitome of sport. It is a contest, a struggle, an agony. Running on the other hand is play. The emotions I feel on the run are quite different from those in the race. Alone I am at peace. I feel confident. There is a loss of the sense of time and place.

The race is systole, where I am active. The run is diastole, where I am passive. The race is complete, the run is open-ended. The race has consequences, the run has none. The differences multiply, and none is trivial.

There is sport and there is play, the race and run, the experience and the esthetic expression of the experience. We have need of both. Racers deprived of play will sooner or later desert their sport. Runners who never compete will move on to other interests, and they and their coaches will wonder why it happened.

It takes both sport and play to make our lives complete.

THE RACE IS A TRUE EXPERIENCE. Only the conditions are artificial. My entire self is engaged in a genuine struggle against time and distance and those around me. All my strengths, physical and emotional and moral, are called upon to decide the issue.

The race is, as Santayana said: "A great and continuing endeavor, a representation of all the primitive virtues and fundamental gifts of man."

Because it involves these primitive virtues and these fundamental gifts, the race is an uplifting event. It tells me previously unrecognized truths about myself. It fills my subconscious with the experience of the "good me." It makes me a hero and floods my innermost life with proof of that fact.

Our highest need is to be a hero. We need heroic experiences to saturate our subconscious, to fill up our psychic reservoir. It is imperative that this "deep well of cerebration," as William James called it, contain good news rather than bad—that what later comes to the surface is positive rather than negative.

But to be a hero, we must find what best allows us to do something heroic. We must find that arena, find that event. In this duel with life, we are allowed to choose our own weapons. We have the right to fight from high ground.

James wrote of this situation in a letter to his wife: "I often thought that the best way to define personal character would be to seek out the particular mental or moral attitude in which, when it came upon him, he felt himself most deeply and intensely active and alive. At such moments, there is a voice inside which speaks and says, 'This is the real me.' "

That is the voice I hear at the race. The race is, for one thing, absolutely true. Everything is seen and felt exactly as it is. The pain is real. The suffering is real. I am challenged. I respond to that challenge. And when I come to the finish line, I am completely spent yet completely happy. I have forgotten momentarily all the bad things about myself.

But the race is more than the moment. The subconscious is being purged and rinsed and cleansed. It is being emptied of all the mean and embarrassing things I have accumulated during my life. My bedrock concept of myself and the world is being refurbished. I am replacing all the depressing memories, all the dirt and debris, with something that is bright and clean and positive. I am hearing the good news.

This is most necessary because the subconscious is the source of all our creativity. Creativity in the arts or in thought or in life situations depends upon a subconscious that contains what is good and true and joyful. It must be kept free of everything that is not.

Hemingway once wrote that he never read criticism of his works because they made his subconscious murky and muddy. And, he said, he had to be kept clean if he was to write.

We don't have to read critics to make our subconscious murky and muddy. All we have to do is go to work, or go to school, or go to church, or even perhaps go home. There are critics all around us. Rarely do we hear anything that would make us feel good about ourselves. Our subconscious is constantly being crammed with evidence of our shortcomings and failures.

The race reverses that. It tells me I am a success. It makes me feel good about myself. And later in the week, this experience percolates out of my subconscious when I am at play—on my training runs, where I am in control, feeling virtuous at an eight-minute-per-mile pace. Then I write my column, or plan my day, or think in new directions—all because of this new "me" that has come into being.

Our problems are solved creatively, or even left unsolved creatively, only by a profound and thorough alteration of our inner life.

The race is my transforming experience. It causes a profound and thorough alteration of my inner life. The training run is the play in which this experience finds its esthetic expression. The experience of the race germinating in my conscious mind comes to fruition in play.

Then the freedom of the body and mind takes the event and its meaning, and produces art—the outer form in which life finds expression and support. Whether this is a poem or a statue, a letter or a garden, a recipe or a relationship, makes little difference. Whatever the expression, it will be a new representation of you when you are deeply and intensely active and alive.

Now you can say, "This is me," and be proud to say it.

Chapter Eighteen
On Motivating

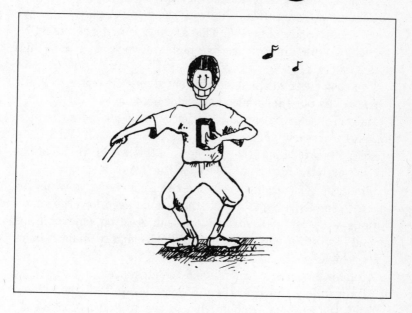

"The common aim of athletes is consistent top-level performance—not longevity, not disease prevention, not health or wellness. Their goal is to play their game well. Whatever helps them do this is worthwhile. . . ."

I DON'T BELIEVE in will power. I believe in *want* power. If you want a thing badly enough you'll do whatever is necessary to obtain it. So it is with exercise. You may just want to run, period, or walk, or swim. Your sport may be an end in itself. Or you may train as a means to something else you want badly. Either way, you develop the want power to make exercise a part of your life.

"I hate running, but I like what it does," says golfer Jack Nicklaus. "If I want to keep up with the younger players, I have to take better care of myself. That's where running comes in."

Nicklaus runs three miles five nights a week at about 8 minutes a mile.

"I just want to get it done without dying," he says. "Oh it's horrible . . . but I feel much better for doing it."

Nicklaus has given running a priority in his life, because it has become necessary for his number one priority—golf. What is at stake is his profession, the way he is in this world. He identifies himself with the way he performs on the links.

When the relationship between exercise and everyday performance is immediate and direct, there is no need for other motivation—no necessity to make exercise interesting, enjoyable and an end in itself. A person is quite willing to find room for it in his daily schedule.

Athletes, especially professional athletes, are willing to make that adjustment. Most of them become aware that their talent will not last without training. If you are an athlete, your body demands athletic care. Diet and exercise, sleep and relaxation, are elements of extreme importance.

Professional basketball players stress the importance of sufficient rest, proper diet and ability to relax. Getting enough sleep is critical.

"In an 82-game season, players' off-court habits can be the difference between winning 15 games or losing them," says Elgin Baylor of the Washington Bullets.

The legendary Bill Russell agrees: "I knew how to relax, and that's probably the most important thing. I was an excellent sleeper."

Phil Jackson, former Knicks star, sees the need for more exercise as well. "I used to run and swim for conditioning," he says. "I'd walk and walk rather than hang around the hotel. I napped about 40 minutes a day for six days a week. Because of these things, there was a marked increase in the productivity of my game. Instead of being erratic, I became consistent."

The common aim of athletes is consistent top-level performance—not longevity, not disease prevention, not health or wellness. Their goal is to play their game well. Whatever helps them do this is worthwhile, however dull and mindless and boring it might be.

Running is a bore to most golfers, yet many have accepted it. "On the PGA tour years ago," says Nicklaus, "no one ran. Now lots of fellows out there run, maybe 50 or 60."

Arnold Palmer is one of them. Observers thought Palmer was on the way to being the stereotyped middle-aged man with a paunch, puffy face, and a penchant for beer and easy chairs. Palmer noticed it, too. "I was getting a little heavy," he says. "My golf wasn't going good. I was getting tired and lethargic about my game. And I'd lost interest in finding out what was wrong and working on it."

Then Palmer turned his life around: "I started running and now run three miles every morning. As a result, I have lost 20 pounds. My disposition has improved. I've got my old stamina back and the patience to iron out the problems of my game."

A fitness program should offer what a person wants and offer it right now. Promises work with some but disillusion others. Professional athletes look for performance. For them, life expectancy is what they expect out of today's game or tomorrow's match. Athletes seek their full potential every working day, not in some future retirement. Athletes want to be living, achieving legends.

Someone asked Jack Nicklaus if he was a reluctant runner.

"Reluctant perhaps," he answered, "but a believer nevertheless. I feel good, I look better, and that's the key to everything."

When the gains are immediate and measurable, these athletes will do almost anything to get them. So will we all.

WHEN PEOPLE TELL ME running is boring, I know what they mean. I find swimming boring. When I have to swim because I've been injured and can't run, I can do it for what seems like a half hour and find that only five minutes have passed. Swimming is as interminable for me as running is for some people.

I am made for running, not swimming. I have low body fat, which is good for a runner, but bad for a swimmer. I lack the buoyancy and insulation that good swimmers need. I tend to sink instead of float, and I have to expend a considerable amount of energy to keep moving. Although my running form is economical, my swimming stroke is awkward and inefficient. I am always shipping water and am never quite sure what to do with my head. How anyone can enjoy swimming is beyond me.

A physical education professor recently wrote to me about his problem with dropouts in his fitness program. "Why do people who seem to be convinced of the value of cardiovascular health stop exercising?" he asked. His own answer was that psycho-social factors are the prime determinants of behavior.

I am not sure what he means by that, but if he means boredom, I agree. The real question was asked a long time ago: "Why do children who love to play hate physical education?" If we knew the answer to that, we would know why adults drop out of fitness programs. My answer is: because the programs are boring.

Still, the educator is on the right track. Fitness programs do succeed when they satisfy psychological and social needs, like Maslow's needs of belonging, esteem and self-actualization. There is little place for reason or logic. Sport, which is play intensified, is the key. It unlocks the enthusiasm and discipline necessary to satisfy these needs.

One of the most successful fitness programs was one developed by Bruno Balke at the University of Wisconsin. When I called and asked him what his method was, he told me I would have to come and observe it. There is no way, he said, that he could systematically outline his program for me.

What he did was treat each person individually. In effect, he had as many fitness programs as there were people attending. He tried to discover an activity that each person enjoyed, and he used exercise leaders who liked people. He turned his classroom into a playground.

Conversation can be the difference between a fitness program that succeeds and one that fails. I have a friend who has a high-pressure job and has been running 2 to 3 miles a day for years. He was originally a physical education teacher and runs for a number of reasons, including fitness and relaxation, but he has never really enjoyed running. He does enjoy, however, the way running makes him feel.

Some months ago another runner moved into his neighborhood. This man is the same build as my friend. He also has the same temperament: gregarious and outgoing. They began to run together, talking all the while. The runs soon extended to 6 and 7 miles a day. Time and distance passed unnoticed. Now they have been joined by a third runner who matches them in style, interests and pace. The trio logs mile after mile, chattering like magpies.

One physical educator began a successful jogging program for dentists using the same device. He discovered that dentists rarely get to speak to other dentists, so his plan allows for a maximum of talk. "We take a long time in the locker room getting dressed," he told me. "Then we jog out to one dentist's house and have danish and coffee. Then we jog back and take a long time getting showered and dressed."

I once spoke at a highly successful fitness clinic in the Midwest run by an outstanding exercise physiologist. Afterward, when his secretary was driving me back to the airport, she confessed that she didn't participate. There was nothing in it she liked to do, she said. I asked her what she did like. "Oh, I love to dance," she told me. "I'm always the last to leave at a dance." Yet this widely imitated clinic did not have a dance program.

"Don't serve time," said bank robber Willie Sutton. "Make time serve you." Fitness programs shouldn't be cruel or unusual punishment. The time spent getting fit should be as interesting and happy as other parts of the day.

ONE LOOK AT THE PROGRAM and I knew the President's Council on Physical Fitness and Sports was taking this meeting seriously. This one-day symposium on "Health and Fitness: The Corporate View" featured all the big guns the council could muster. They had brought in experts from all over the country. The hotel register read like a *Who's Who* in health, fitness and preventive medicine.

I was there in a nonscientific capacity. Such events tend to get too serious and even a little tedious. The participants need a little diversion. I was one diversion. George Allen, the ex-football coach, was another. The Marine Corps Band was a third. Allen was to speak at the luncheon. The band and I drew the dinner.

Allen's talk followed a morning of lectures on fitness and life expectancy, fitness and disease prevention medicine, fitness and coronary risk factors, fitness and absenteeism. The afternoon promised more of the same. The same weapons, the same ammunition, the same claims of success.

All the while I knew something was missing. This fusillade of graphs and charts and statistics, I was sure, had no more moved the audience than it had moved me. I was reminded of Napoleon's comment about the cavalry charge: "It's magnificent, but it's not war."

What we were being told had everything but relevance. There was nothing that would cause the people in board rooms to conscript their troops and ready them for battle.

I thought then of Nietzsche's statement. "Once you know 'Why,' " he said, "you will accept any 'How.' " We had yet to hear a compelling "Why," yet to be told something that would spur these executives into joining this campaign for fitness.

Then George Allen gave his speech. It was untitled, but it became immediately evident it was about winning. Allen is himself a winning coach and a winning speaker. Short declarative sentences with plenty of bite: that's the Allen style. Ideas that illuminate you and the task before you. Fifteen minutes of Allen and you can't wait for the game to start. You can't wait for adversity to begin.

He told of his experience with the Washington Redskins. "We took that over-the-hill gang," he said, "and out-conditioned every team in the league." The Redskins, old as they were, became the best fourth-quarter team in football. And they did it by following Allen's rules for becoming a winner.

None of these rules is new. They go back to the Book of Genesis. And they are as American as apple pie and mother. Allen is pure Emerson. He expresses the philosophy of people in process, reaching for perfection. So he told us nothing new, forcefully. Oh, so forcefully, he told us what we had forgotten. Again and again he came back to those pioneer virtues. Work hard. Stick together. Have the right attitude. Be positive. Improve every day. And always ask the question, "How badly do I want it?" The other teams don't beat you, said Allen. You beat yourself.

What it came down to, said Allen, was winning. For the athlete winning was the goal, the applause, a new birth, the fruit of the harvest. Winning was the best getting better. And it began and ended with conditioning. There was no substitute for physical fitness.

The band opened the dinner that night. I was to close it. The Marines contributed some stirring songs, reaching a climax with "America, the Beautiful," and closing with hymns of the various services. Now I had to put the day in focus. I was to say something that would move these executives to action, somehow induce them to take the idea of fitness and make it a reality.

During my introduction I suddenly realized what I had to say. I put my prepared talk aside, and told them the truth. And the truth was that the best thing they had heard all day was George Allen and the Marine Corps band. They had appealed to something higher and of infinitely more value than the medical rewards offered by the experts.

Corporations are engaged in competition as fierce as any encountered in the National Football League. And there is a continual corporate Olympics vying with corporations in other countries as well. Fitness can make a company a winner. Fitness is no longer a luxury; it is a necessity.

They had heard the Gospel according to George Allen. I would merely give the exegesis. "Do you," I asked them, "have the best fourth-quarter corporation in your industry? Are you coaching, training, prodding your corporate team to do its best? Have you out-conditioned the rest of your league?

"Forget longevity, heart attacks, disease prevention, absenteeism," I told them. "They have nothing to do with fitness. Besides, what is longevity to you? Of what benefit is it to the corporation if someone lives to be eighty? And there must be dozens of employees you wish would have a mild heart attack so you could replace them. And what about absenteeism? Figures show that 90 percent of absenteeism is due to 10 percent of the work force. Pick your employees like a football coach. 'Give me men,' said Lombardi, 'not players. Players are a dime a dozen.'

"Corporations are a dime a dozen, too. Think of building a winning corporation," I urged them, "filled with people capable of increased work and more production. Employees and the company then take on the same personality. They become a single entity. Winning employees make for a winning corporation. If you would have a company with energy and enthusiasm and imagination, your employees must have the same qualities."

This was important not only to the employees and to corporations, it was important to the country. America will win this corporate international war, this conflict of energy, creativity and productivity, only if each individual employee can make that identical contribution of energy, creativity and productivity.

It ended there. The symposium was over. The band was packing up the instruments. The executives were filing out. Had they decided to take action? It did not matter. In time they would have to. Even now people are doing it on their own, seeing fitness as an obligation, a personal responsibility.

I sat there still high on Allen's words and the Marine Band's music. I was, I realized, very bullish on Americans. We are in a contest where class will tell. At that moment, I was sure we had it.

Chapter Nineteen
On Psyching

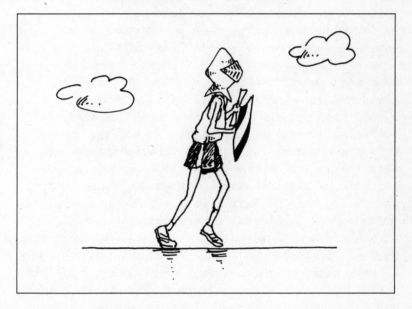

"Motivation, whether it be in poetry or prizefighting, must come from deep within. We cannot expect to find it in a life that is completely rational. What we need is passion. Passion alone enables us to face up to and even revel in stress."

IN AN ADDRESS to the American Philosophical Society, William James took as his theme "The Energies of Man." He had been musing for many years, he told his colleagues, on the phenomenon of the second wind. He had observed that there was even a third wind and a fourth wind. He saw, he said, evidence of reserves of energy that we rarely called upon.

"The plain fact remains," he said, "that men the world over possess amounts of resources that only exceptional individuals push to their extremes of use." Compared to what we ought to be, he told his fellow philosophers, we are only half-awake. We have powers of various sorts we habitually fail to use.

James's purpose that night more than 75 years ago was to consider two questions: First, to what extent do we have energies? Second, what are the keys to unlocking them?

These questions are characteristic of James. He was himself a restless, driven person. He was obsessed with the problem of the energies of man—the thoroughly American problem of how to get the most out of yourself.

America is an affluent society, and now that we have the time and money to be anything we can be, the answers to the questions propounded by James seem more important.

To what extent, then, do we have energies? The almost awesome energies posited by James in the common man are rapidly becoming visible as more and more ordinary human beings turn to distance running. Millions of people are running. Hundreds of thousands enter weekly races where the most popular distance is a previously incredible 10 kilometers. Thousands upon thousands complete the marathon and runs longer than 26 miles, 385 yards.

This is not merely a movement of men at their physiological peak. These millions include people of all ages, and between 20 and 30 percent of them are women. There seems to be no limit to the endurance of young and middle-aged and elderly men and women.

What has happened is that people have become athletes and, in so doing, have discovered previously unsuspected energies that James said were there on demand.

What are the keys to unlocking these energies? James saw

that as our primary question, the problem of motivation. What is it that impels this move to be all that is possible?

"To what," James mused, "do these men owe their escape?"

The answer, he thought, was excitement, ideas and efforts. We must discover in the social realm something that demands incredible efforts, depth beyond depth of exertions both in degree and duration. We need something heroic that will cut across all class and economic divisions. We need incitements and passions and enthusiasms. We need to give our word of honor. Any or all of these might do.

Sport does all that. Sport motivates the athlete. It is something that demands supreme effort. It is something heroic that speaks to all, something with built-in incitements and passions and enthusiasms.

I saw the questions asked by James answered clearly on a visit I made to West Point. I was taken on a tour of the gymnasium, where I saw hundreds of cadets engaged in all sorts of sports. "There are more calories expended a day in this gym," said my escort, "than in most moderate-sized cities." Later in the captain's office I saw a motto on the wall that told the story. "Every student, an athlete. For every athlete, a challenge." Once we find our sport, we become athletes. "Those secular saints," James called them. Just as he called saints "the athletes of God." Sport provides the challenge, the impetus, the motivation. It becomes the purifying discipline.

In closing his address, James suggested that human beings be studied with reference to the different ways in which their energy reserve may be released.

Present-day philosophers and investigators of human potential might begin by stopping the next runner they see on the road. People who are tapping their deeper resources are no longer the exception. There are millions who are experiencing an escape to their high selves. Most of them are athletes. Many of them are runners.

WHEN PETER MORGAN WAS coaching track at Princeton, I asked him about the progress of a freshman runner I knew. "He's running well," Morgan replied, "but I'm afraid we may lose him. He's a thinker.

"When a runner gets back to the dorm, someone usually asks him, 'Why are you knocking yourself out? Why go through that torture?' If the runner is a thinker, he begins to think about that and frequently fails to come up with a good answer. Then he quits."

The young runner did quit. He had learned all about stress and how to handle it, how to condition his body, and how to minimize the bad effects. He had learned how to relax and how to recuperate. He'd been taught how much his body could take and how to recognize danger signs. The coach had taught him all that. What he did not learn, and could not be taught, was the "Why?" That had to come from himself.

We all have an inner voice asking: "Why am I trying so hard? Why am I knocking myself out?" Man is a maximizer, pursuing ease or hardship, pleasure or pain with equal intensity. We can direct all our energies into making life easy, or we can undergo the worst sufferings to achieve an ideal. We are willing to take on hand-to-hand struggle or minute-by-minute, day-by-day conflict with ourselves only if we know why we are doing it. The German philosopher Friedrich Nietzsche, as we have observed, told us that if we have a why to live, we will also find a how.

Philosopher William James addressed this topic in his speech, "What Makes a Life Significant." The answer, he said, was the marriage of an unhabitual ideal with some fidelity, courage and endurance. When that miracle occurs, we not only accept stress, we welcome it.

The poet John Berryman said much the same thing. "What happens to my poetic work in the future," he said, "will not depend upon my sitting calmly on my ass, but by my being knocked in the face and thrown flat and given all sorts of illnesses short of senile dementia." Poet Marianne Moore, speaking of former heavyweight boxing champion Floyd Patterson, said his motivation was a matter of "powerful feeling and the talent to use it."

Such motivation, whether it be in poetry or prizefighting, must come from deep within. We cannot expect to find it in a life that is completely rational. What we need is passion. Passion alone enables us to face up to and even revel in stress. What is necessary is a cause, an experience, a value, even some suffering that will enflame us, not just for a moment, but continuously.

That is another difficulty. Anyone can get fired up for a while, because most of us have ideals. We all wish, but we don't always have the desire or the ambition required to make our wishes happen. We don't really want to change the world; we'd rather go down to the corner and have a beer.

The need still exists, however, for a continuing ideal, a persistent value for which we will live, love and fight during every waking hour—some meaning for which we would be willing to die. That is the paradox.

But how do we find such motivation? How do we begin this search for meaning? One way is to face up to psychiatrist Viktor Frankl's question to the despairing patient: "Why not, then, commit suicide?"

Why don't we? Because faced with that choice we begin to see what we want. We realize that our life has meaning, that we can leave a mark, and the world will be aware that we were here.

One way to do this, as the poet Robert Frost suggested, is to achieve form. It matters little, he said, what form it is. A basket, a letter, a garden, a room, an idea, a picture, a poem would do. This is the artist's view. Inspiration followed by perspiration. Passion followed by precision.

Whatever we do must be preceded by our will to achieve; the will to search for these things and then be committed to accomplishing them.

The thinker, as Coach Morgan said, is always in danger. We athletes who tend to be thinkers, rather than doers or talkers, know that. But once we see the light, there is nothing we won't do to reach it.

IF THERE IS A RACE I should avoid, it is the Trevira Twosome. It comes only six days after the Boston Marathon, hardly time to recoup for a 10-miler on Central Park's toughest course—10 miles of rolling hills and a finish that is a long, steady upgrade to the Tavern on the Green. The Trevira is an hour-plus of unremitting pain—a continuous, desperate but losing effort to keep up with the flow, with little to show for it. My performance at the Trevira never reflects its cost.

Yet each year I stand there with thousands of others, waiting for the starter's gun—all of us impatient to get on with this challenge. Many of us are still hurting from Boston but oblivious to everything else in our lives, completely focused on the race ahead.

Why do we do it? What is there that brings us out week after week in cities and towns all over the country to run these races? Why do we make such demands on our bodies, endure such hardship, go through so much pain?

When Prince Charles, no stranger to arduous and even dangerous activities, was asked why people do such things, he had an answer: "I call it the banging-your-head-against-the-wall syndrome. It feels so good when you stop. But more than that, it makes you appreciate things you have always taken for granted."

The race is a superior way to bang your head against the wall. It is a contest with yourself more than others.

"A contest," writes the philosopher Paul Weiss, "demands that one complete a task. It rarely provides pleasure or fun." The primary emphasis in a distance run, says Weiss, is on struggle and self-discovery.

Three minutes into the Trevira, it is already a struggle. I am totally occupied in maintaining a speed that is just too fast for my chest and arms and legs. I am seeking some compromise between pace and pain. And all the while, I am being passed by a horde of fellow runners.

In those three minutes, I have left an effortless existence and entered one where I am pushing my life supports to the limit.

"The healthy body lives in silence," writes Alexis Carrel. "You cannot hear it, you cannot feel it. Inside deep is the whir of a 16-cylinder motor, and from deep within comes a harmony and peace."

I have left that peace and harmony. That silence has been shattered. I have become a gasping, groaning caricature of the runner who had stood quietly awaiting the gun.

The miles pass without letup. A hill comes, and the groans get louder. Everything temporarily gets worse. I feel the vicelike grip of lactic acid on my legs. My breathing, already inadequate, goes to 60 a minute, and still my whole body is screaming for more air. I am banging my head against the wall and feeling every bang.

I look at my watch. This eternity has lasted 52 minutes. I know then that it will go on for another 12 minutes or more. I have a little less than two miles of suffering left. I have done that innumerable times and know I can do it again—no matter what lies ahead.

I remember I have done it before. But I forgot how terrible it was in the doing. What I have done is only prologue. Now the attrition of those 10 miles, the fatigue and the exhaustion will be added to the pain that has gone on before.

In that last mile I am no more than an animal struggling to reach safety. I am using resources, strength and will and endurance that human beings mobilize only in life-threatening situations. I am reaching for the innermost core that is "I" and no one else—the "I" who is my truth, the isolated essence below and beneath any other "I" that I ever knew.

Somehow I reach that last quarter-mile. I come to that infamous uphill finish and I try to run faster, to pick up my pace. I am running as fast as I can, head back, arms grasping the air. The legs become stiffer and stiffer, heavier and heavier. I am stabbing at the ground. I can't hang on any longer. My body is saying no more, no more, and then I am in the chute. The race is over. The banging has ceased.

It is as Prince Charles has said. It does feel good when I stop. The pain is already subsiding. The breathing has become manageable. The warmth is coming back to my body. I have come back to what was all there at the starting line: a world and a life and friends I took for granted. No longer.

I am now, as the French say, engaged. I do not look; I see. I do not touch; I feel. I do not smell; I scent. I do not taste; I savor.

The sunlight has become precious, the breeze a delight. What I was blind to, I now see plain. I know the meaning in a handshake, the treasure in a smile. Being alive has become a mystical experience.

As I lie there on the grass, I know the Kingdom of Heaven is already here.

Chapter Twenty
On
Inspiring

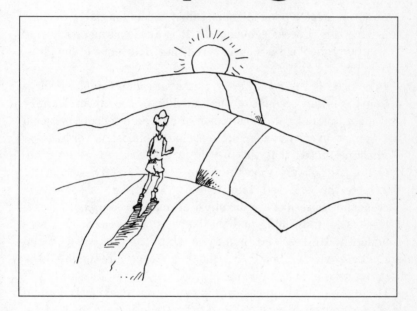

"I am increasingly aware that I know more
than I can tell. Much of that knowledge
comes from my body. It is the body more
than anything else that contributes to my
feelings of certainty, or self-control, or self-
esteem."

"AT ONE TIME, one of the aims of my mind was to know how a man with a massive physique felt about the world around him," wrote Yukio Mishima in *Sun and Steel*, his psychological autobiography. "Then suddenly I was the one with the fine physique."

Mishima, the man of words, had finally become his own body. He had learned what came to be his second language, the language of the flesh.

Sun and Steel, a book Mishima called "a confidential criticism," tells how this process came about. It is a fascinating account of how a puny, bookish boy discovered the importance of his physical being.

It is also, as the book jacket points out, an attempt to relate action to art; an account of one individual's search for identity and integrity and a demonstration of how an intensely personal preoccupation can develop into a profound philosophy of life.

Mishima states that this revolutionary change occurred because of his pondering on the nature of the "I." These meditations on the self led him to the conclusion that the "I" corresponded precisely to the physical space he occupied. He saw his self as the dwelling and the body as the orchard that surrounded it. He resolved then to cultivate the orchard with sun and steel—the sun being the cult of the open air, the steel the weights used in body building.

He entered a new phase in his education. Previously he had concentrated on his genius in writing. He did not understand reality and action and the flesh. Now that had all changed. He was following the guidelines set out by the Greeks, the *paideia*. This was no less than a lifelong process of transformation. The *paideia* was not merely learning; it was the making and shaping of the man himself as a work of art.

The steel led to that transformation in Mishima. It made him a work of art.

"By its subtle, infinitely varied operation," he wrote, "the steel restored the classic balance the body had begun to lose—reinstating it in its natural form, the form it should have had all along."

Muscles seem useless and irrelevant in modern life. They are usually unnecessary from a practical point of view. Mishima admitted this. However, they gave him an entirely new kind of knowledge—a knowledge that neither books nor experience could impart.

William James, in his *Gospel of Relaxation*, thought that muscular vigor also corresponded to the spirit. It lent, he said, a background of sanity, serenity and good humor.

Once into his body, Mishima never looked back. He turned to fencing and then to running. Running was a mystery. "It washed away the emotions of the daily round," he reported. "Before long, my blood would not permit me a halt of even a day or two. Something ceaselessly set me to work. My body would no longer tolerate indolence but began instantly to thirst for violent action, urging me on."

His life then became what observers must have considered a frenzied obsession. "My solace," he declared, "lay solely in the small rebirths of the soul and flesh that occurred immediately after the exercise."

It was in the exercise and these rebirths that Mishima found the touchstone of the writer, the ability to translate reality into words. So he did not come back reluctantly to the world of words. These rebirths of the soul and the flesh ensured that he could return to writing joyfully and with a glad heart.

I know this to be true, as I return time and time again from my encounters with my body. When I run, my body is the Good Me. I experience it in a unique and genuine way of knowing that includes perception as well as verbalization.

Running has given me a physical intelligence, a biological wisdom. Previously I was deaf to the body's signals, blind to its illuminations. The body, I have discovered, has a mind of its own.

Other cultures have always known this. There is a Zen saying that in the dark the mind is in the fingers. There was also an Indian chief who once told Carl Jung why white men had wrinkled faces: "They think only with their heads."

I am increasingly aware that I know more than I can tell. Much

‫‪...‬‬at knowledge comes from my body. It is the body more than anything else that contributes to my feelings of certainty, or self-control, or self-esteem.

When I began running, I was 160 pounds. Now I am 136 pounds, my running weight in college. I now occupy the right amount of space. I move with ease and grace and endurance.

Where Mishima became the classic weight lifter, I have become the classic distance runner. Where his body possessed certain qualities, mine possesses others. I too have seen the correspondence between the body and the spirit. But it is my body and my spirit, no other. And it is my intensely individual preoccupation with running that has developed my philosophy in life.

There are times when the all-powerful intellect is only an interpreter, and a poor one at that. It continues to seek truth as the soul seeks the good. The self desires all this and more. The fully functioning and knowing and loving self desires action and sweat and the total use of a playful body.

Mishima said it all: Become the athlete your body has to be.

"SHARED SUFFERING," wrote Yukio Mishima in *Sun and Steel* "is the ultimate nonverbal expression." The pain we undergo with others takes us to an area where language fails and silence begins. It was just that area which Mishima sought. *Sun and Steel* is an odyssey of an artist of the word, a man of surpassing genius in verbal imagery, seeking the representation of experience in purer form. That ultimate expression he found in group pain. In that special union with others, he joined art and action.

He began by becoming an athlete. His body, he discovered, spoke a language of its own. It did not speak Japanese. Next came pain—not the vicarious pain of the writer, but the real and actual proof of consciousness that athletes undergo. And then he underwent that most difficult of conversions for an intellectual and an artist: he became a member of a group.

He came to realize that the use of strength and the ensuing fatigue, the sweat and the blood, could confer the glorious sense of being the same as the others. And so, in the final scene of this book, we see him running in the dim light of morning—one of a group, stripped to the waist in the freezing air.

"Through the common suffering," he tells us, "the shared cries of encouragement and the chorus of voices, I felt the slow emergence, like the sweat that gradually beaded my skin, of the affirmation of identity, of nobility, of being united in seeking death and glory."

Every athlete might not put it quite so dramatically, but athletes know that what Mishima writes is true. My own life as a runner has duplicated his personal journey—first becoming an athlete, then feeling the pain and finally reaching the race. I came to running and became my body. I took to the roads and felt pain. Then I went into the race and knew that here was something unlike any other relationship I had ever had.

Mishima saw that. The group, he contended, has a special language. "Whether it is written down on paper or shouted aloud," he writes, "the language of the group resolves itself into physical expression." This is not the speech of the solitary artist. Mishima the writer knew that. "This is not a language," he says, "for transmitting private messages from the solitude of one's closed room to the solitude of another distant closed room."

The group is concerned with all those things that could never emerge in words: sweat and tears, joy and pain.

"Verbal expression can convey pleasure or grief; it cannot convey pain," writes Mishima. "Only bodies placed under the same circumstances can experience a common suffering."

Unamuno, the Spanish philosopher, makes the same point: "We are united by pity, not by pleasure. We love only those with whom we share suffering." There can be no love without pain.

All of that is felt during the race. And at the finish words again fail us. It is the race itself that is our language. The running is the word made flesh. The group and the suffering speak within each of us. We have been united in a way words can never accomplish.

Each runner in a race contributes suffering and pain and previously unknown energies to a common cause. The race unites the one and the many. It illuminates the paradox of remaining an individual yet identifying with a group.

"I belonged to them," he writes, "they belonged to me; the two formed an unmistakable 'us.' " It was the beginning, he notes, of his placing reliance on others—a reliance that was mutual.

In the race, I feel this same belonging, develop this same trust, come to this same faith. So the race becomes for me what running that morning was for Mishima: "A bridge that once crossed left no means for return."

AFTER I BECAME INTERESTED in Yukio Mishima's *Sun and Steel*, a friend questioned me about it.

"I don't know how you can read Mishima," she said. "He was obsessed with death."

She was absolutely right. Mishima was so preoccupied with death that he described life as a rehearsal for his death. *Sun and Steel* makes that evident. In a real sense, this book is a suicide note. In November 1970, the year it was published, Mishima committed *seppuku*—ritual suicide.

To Mishima, the process of becoming his total self, his own perfection, meant becoming uncompromisingly and unendingly the person he conceived himself to be. Mishima was one of those people we regard with amazement. They do not have views; they are views. They do not have opinions; they live them. They do not write about theories; they make them realities. They do not talk about myths; they act them out. They are the heroes.

Mishima was a hero. This does not mean that he was right or rational or to be commended for what he did. It does mean that he lived what he believed. In the course of that life, he did things that were childish and foolish and, from our point of view, incomprehensible. All his decisions and judgments came from inside himself. He was interested in nothing but the ideal life that he had set in front of himself.

Like most heroes, Mishima imposed his will on reality. And further, he saw his will as the will of the universe. He became body-mind-soul the creature he believed his Creator had in mind the day he was born.

No matter how illogical and irrational it may seem to praise this man's book, *Sun and Steel* is filled with wisdom and common sense. Mishima was much like a person with paranoia. Aside from his single delusion, his life was completely sane. Aside from his obsession, his book reads as a text on how to become and develop and love your self. He expressed this union of mind and spirit as few had done before him.

One reason for this is that he came upon the body from another culture. He saw its perfection in much the same way a man blind from birth suddenly sees the world. *Sun and Steel* is no ordinary book on the role of the body in this life, not just another volume of the effect of sport and play on man. It is a testimony by the most ardent of lovers, the truest of believers, the convert who came last to the faith.

I have come to accept Mishima's truth. His "steel" is my running. His discovery of the body parallels my own. Where he translated his intensely individual interest into a philosophy of death, I have been able to translate mine into a philosophy of life.

Mishima modeled his life on a great myth, not a petty success story. He lived the questions and did not wait for answers. He showed the tremendous intensity and enthusiasm we need, and how large a canvas we must use, if life is to take on meaning.

Chapter Twenty-One
On
Thinking

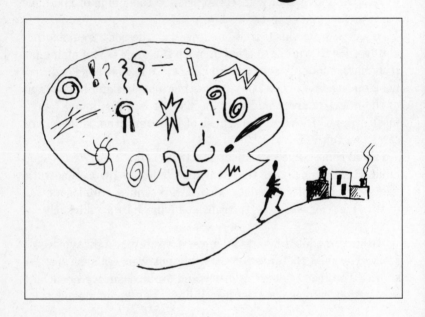

"The athletic life is as mental as it is physical.
Training becomes so automatic that the
mind is free to do whatever it pleases. The
muscles need no conscious direction, so the
mind can occupy center stage."

I RECEIVED A PHONE CALL from a man whose son was in trouble in college. This young man had written an essay on "Positive Addiction" describing his experiences as an oarsman on the freshman crew. From what I could see, it was something I had read many times: a recounting of the conversion phenomenon which so many people go through in becoming athletes.

Unfortunately, his professor was unaware of this universal human reaction. He happened to read William Glasser's *Positive Addiction* and assumed that the student had cribbed his theme and material from this book—a book, incidentally, that was written by runners as much as by Glasser. Glasser solicited personal testimony of the running experience from readers of *Runner's World*, and the book was the outcome of those letters. The student says he never read the book. I believe him.

Here, in effect, was simply another contribution to that book. Rather than being inspired by the book, it was very like one of those personal stories from which it was made. The new insight, new life, new sense of self that this freshman presented in his essay were indubitably his own.

I recall in school that the use of the word "I" was discouraged. The personal was too trivial to consider. If one is to be educated, that education must be left to the experts. We were not allowed to live out our own lives or, even more, to consider them important. The common man, despite the influence of Emerson and Thoreau and James, was considered a cipher.

What I see in the indictment of this oarsman is the continuation of that attitude. I would suggest to this professor that he reread his Emerson about the common man. Emerson writes, "What Plato thought, he can think. What the saint felt, he can feel. What happened to any man, he can understand." And then again, "The philosopher spends his life putting into words what the common man experiences."

Long ago, I called a five-mile run "a trip" and suggested it was an addiction, a fix if you would. Long before Glasser, I read a speech by Edwin Land, the inventor of the Polaroid camera, saying that we are all addicts of something. What we need, said Land, are constructive addictions, not destructive ones. That was my first contact with the idea of positive addiction, and I wrote about it in my column six or seven years ago.

All runners have known this addiction, and many of them have tried to put it in much the same words. Any editor of a running magazine can tell you of being deluged by stories which their writers presume to be original, but which are almost the same.

There are only a few truths, a few themes. There is so little to write about. The even greater truth is that these truths occur to everyone and that there are those of us who burn to write them just as if we were geniuses.

I doubt my gift for writing. To further limit any loss of self-esteem, I rarely read live writers. I look on them as competition. I do not want to be derivative. Yet I find myself taking the same theme and frequently using the same words. How can this be?

One answer would be the inadequacy of language. No two individuals, no two experiences, are exactly alike. Yet we cannot express that uniqueness without also expressing its similarity to something else. We cannot make it stand alone. If this young man failed in his essay, it is because everyone fails. No one can tell us exactly why it is different for him. Therefore, in the telling, he tells us what we have ourselves experienced but have never been able to say either. So it lies there between us, almost right but not quite, almost true but not quite.

For those outside the experience, the whole thing is a mystery. Not knowing the truth, they cannot see what went on inside the person and cannot know—however stereotyped the presentation—that it is as true and accurate as one's genius permits.

The athletic experience will be forever a mystery to those who have forgotten their childhood and never again suspect that the good life has its roots in the perfection of the human body.

TRAIN YOUR BRAIN and your body at the same time.

This is not a new idea. It goes back to the original philosophers in Greece who found their best thoughts while walking and thereby attending to their physical fitness. One reads of this phenomenon again and again in the journals of the great thinkers and writers and artists. They were often great walkers as well.

Not only can one train the body while one is using the mind; the mind actually works better when the body is in motion. Take 90 minutes a day, and use half of it or more for a walk or a run or a cycle or a swim. Then come back and put the products of your brain's activity on paper or on canvas or into some new appreciation of your life.

In the beginning, both body and mind will balk. When that happens, force the mind back time and again to consider the subject in question. Whatever you have decided to meditate on before you leave the house, require the brain to consider it. The brain is tireless. Do not let it con you into relaxing your demands. Push it to the limit.

The body, too, will say, "That's enough for today." In the beginning, as with the brain, it will want its own way. Don't give in. Make the effort comfortable as possible, but don't stop or turn back. Each day, ask a little more. In a short time, your work capacity can increase as much as 400 percent.

First develop the capabilities for greater physical and mental effort, then decide what to do with them.

IT WAS LATE in the question-and-answer period I usually conduct after my lectures when a man stood up and asked, "What do you think about when you are running?"

I liked the question; it made me think. Most questions are routine. They generate routine answers. They stimulate a reflex arc in my brain and produce an automatic response. Partly this is my fault. Every question has something novel about it. There are an infinite variety of people in an infinite variety of situations. The good teacher—and questions are a good teaching device—should always be alert to the lesson in each one of them.

This question broke new ground. I had never before systematized what went on in my mind when I ran. Yet the athletic life is as mental as it is physical. Training becomes so automatic that the mind is free to do whatever it pleases. The muscles need no conscious direction, so the mind can occupy center stage.

How, then, to use this hour of thought? The question opens up the full range of the mind's activities. I can, should I want to, utilize any of the special skills the mind has. For this hour, I can train my mind to perform new feats as I simultaneously bring my body to a higher level of function.

As he stood there, my mind was leaping to categories. I realized my thinking had become mundane. With all the possibilities out there, I had largely limited myself to two basic uses of that training during my 10-mile runs. With rare exceptions, my runs involve either free association or are focused on one subject, one problem that I would like to solve before I get back to home base.

The exceptions are the days when my goal is complete absence of thought and all external and internal stimuli are gradually removed from consciousness. Motion becomes my mantra. Through it I gradually divest myself of worry and anger, of fear and depression—and the reasons for them. I can reach a state when time is this never-ending moment and where this place is the entire world. This is the passive meditation of the East. The Self subsumed in the Whole.

There is another type of meditation which is active, involving fantasy and imagination. Psychiatrists sometimes recommend it. When you thrust yourself into such a prescribed setting, the ensuing feelings and events help to reveal your psychological problems.

I never practice it. I have poor visual memory, and only with difficulty can I conjure up the undulating green meadows, the landscapes and vistas that are recommended. I prefer to deal with the thoughts and ideas and concepts that come, invited or not, into my mind.

In fact, that may be the best answer to the question of what I think about when I run: simply whatever pops into my brain. I suit up, go out on the run, and there I meet these unexpected ideas and new insights. The old wine in new bottles. It is all unpremeditated. I know this happens with other runners.

Dr. Thomas Tutko, the sports psychologist, speaks of the same experience. "I can't wait to get out on the roads," he says, "to find out what I'm going to think about." It is all as unplanned, as undirected and as unexpected as that.

I have days when that is true. I come upon an interesting topic and explore it for a while. The hour becomes a stream of consciousness, with one tenuously related idea following another. One thought will suggest the next, and as the association goes on, words and people and events are coupled like so many freight trains, each from different railroad lines and different parts of the country.

Then there are days when I discipline my mind to concentrate on one particular theme. My mind still tends, as it does on other days, to go romping off following other leads. But I bring it back as I would a bird dog who wanted to play instead of hunt. And so the hour passes as I focus this 10-billion cell computer in my skull on the problem at hand.

Mental training can be as exciting and varied as physical training. Both are an act of discovery.

Chapter Twenty-two
On
Creating

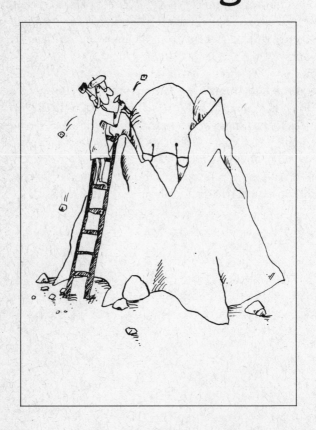

"If the opera is loud and unintelligible and
interminable, get up and leave. Your art is
not there."

IN MY EARLY TEENS I was taken by my aunt, a music teacher, to a performance of *Aïda*. The evening was interminable. Opera, I discovered, was a long, loud and unintelligible bore. I could not wait for it to end so we could head home.

In subsequent exposure to capital "A" Art in other forms, I have had the same reaction. I do not have any grasp or appreciation of what constitutes culture. This is not from lack of trying. I have gone to the Whitney and the Guggenheim museums, sat through concerts at Carnegie Hall, and attended the ballet at Lincoln Center. For all that was happening to my mind and emotions, I might just as well have been riding the subway.

This intimidation by Art disappeared when I became an athlete. I lost the inferiority I felt in the presence of Art, the opera and classical music, painting or the dance. I had discovered the true art, the art of living.

This realization came with a reversal of my role of accepting other people's opinions to one of living my own. The development of the self which occurs with physical training led to that self-expression which I came to recognize as art.

Each one of us is animal, artist, hero, saint. In each of those aspects we have certain abilities and certain disabilities. I knew almost from the first that I would never be the heavyweight boxing champion of the world. What I did not know was that a symphony would never be more to me than a series of pleasant or unpleasant sounds. Nor did I realize that music appreciation was of consequence only to those who appreciated music. I could live long and well and artistically without it.

We have what E. F. Schumaker called "adequatio" for certain mental processes. We are born with them or without them. The knowledge and acceptance of such unchangeable qualities in our makeup can free us to get on with our true vocation, and to such avocations as contribute to the personality that is potential in each of us.

Emerson, my best friend, put me straight in this. "Each individual soul is such," he said, "in virtue of its being able to transform the world into some particular language of its own—if not into a picture or statue or a dance, then into a trade, an art, a science, a mode of living, a character, an influence."

Being an artist is simply discovering the self and then expressing that self in self-chosen terms. Running opened up to me that self and that expression. I found my language. I expressed myself through my body and what I wrote and what I did. No matter that Art is still as unintelligible to me as Chinese.

There is, I now see, an art to everything. There is an art of medicine, an art of selling, an art of child raising. James describes well the art of teaching. It is, he said, the interposition of an imaginative mind between a fact and a pupil. So it is with any art in life.

In a humane society, said Santayana, everything is art. Manners, clothes, politics, conversation. We go around all day being artists if we would but know it. It is difficult at first to see that all my life is an art. Yet every time I read the great thinkers I find this said again and again.

We must express what Emerson called our particular genius. My experiences in both my conscious and subconscious mind are translated into my own individual language. Does this seem too ordinary, too commonplace to be art? Not so. I am now aware of what Ortega called "the wonders of the simple unhaloed hour." I see life face to face and deal with it. I try to put my stamp on every minute and hour and day I live.

So I let my upwardly mobile friends acquire culture and attend the Arts. For those with the "adequatio" to understand and appreciate what they hear and see, this is both a privilege and pleasure. For others it is a waste of time and even a life. They should be in pursuit of their own art and become masters of it.

If the opera is loud and unintelligible and interminable, get up and leave. Your art is not there.

THE DAY EVENTUALLY DAWNS when the fact of your age also dawns on you. You discover you are getting old. Physically certainly, creatively to a degree, and mentally quite perceptibly you are going downhill. "Can it be," you ask yourself, "that I have already lived?"

The age varies. Maybe thirty for the fortunate ones. Fifty for most. For Arnold Bennett it was forty. For John Stuart Mill it was twenty-one. But sooner or later we put to ourselves the old questions concerning the intrinsic value of life. What have I got out of it? What am I likely to get out of it? What's it worth?

The urgency for answers increases when you get older. For the first time you see death approaching. The dying and its attendant urgency make the answer easier. Once dying is accepted, you see the overwhelming importance of each day, the futility of living in the past, the absurdity of living in the future. Living now is life itself.

Countless philosophers grasped that truth, reminding us again and again that we must perceive the folly of neglecting to savor the present, the folly of assuming the future will be any different from the present, the fatuity of dying before we have begun to live.

This does not preclude change. It presupposes it. If this is to be our last day on earth imagine how you would spend it. Yet each day could be that final day—or even the hereafter. "Today," said Lewis Mumford, "may be a fair sample of eternity."

No matter how many philosophers have instructed us in how this day should be spent, each person must test it for himself; each person must be a philosopher. We have a protective and profound egoism that prevents us from accepting ready-made answers. What is it to us what Plato thought unless it agrees with our own experience?

We need not read Plato to realize how little we are doing with our potential. What limited ideas we have about our physical and creative and mental capabilities. How little we accomplish with the marvelous powers we have.

So the first use of this sensation of aging is to break with the past. Life must be a process, a continual movement in word and in thought, the expression of our particular genius. That death lies at the end should not deter us; it should lend impetus.

Some see this process as tragedy. André Malraux wrote that it takes sixty years of incredible effort to make an individual and then he is good only for dying. The late Ernest Becker states this dilemma even more precisely. "A person spends years coming into his own," he wrote, "developing his talent, his unique gifts, perfecting his discrimination, broadening and sharpening his appetite, learning to bear the disappointments of life, becoming mature and seasoned—finally a unique creature in nature standing with some dignity and nobility and transcending the human condition; no longer driven, no longer a complete reflex, not stamped out of any mold . . . and then has to go the way of the grasshopper."

Age as they describe it is the culmination of life. In these observations I do not see tragedy, but hope; not an end, but a goal; not discouragement, but incentive. When we feel aged we are receiving the word not about what we are doing right but what we are doing wrong. We need not, indeed we should not, and will not deteriorate physically and mentally and creatively. We should, as these writers have written, grow in wisdom and will and character. Every day I live can add to the person I am. It is my duty to make that happen.

"YOU LEARN TO USE EVERYTHING that happened in your life, in creating the character you're working on," said Marlon Brando speaking about acting. "You learn to dip into your unconsciousness and make use of every experience you ever had."

I can find no better description of art and creativity. When my life is the work of art, I am creating a character—myself. And I am doing it out of everything I have ever experienced. I am dredging into my unconscious, bringing up everything down to the seaweed.

I am not a motor genius or a mental genius or a creative genius. I am not a spiritual genius. Yet I have what Emerson called my peculiar genius, my personality, which is the sum of those attributes. And no less than Marlon Brando or Picasso or Nureyev or any athlete, artist, hero, saint, I can fulfill that genius. I can become a character and create the self that I am.

Such creativity, says Bill Moyers, who has made a study of the subject, demands that one remain a perpetual child. What creativity demands, it seems to me, is that we have passion. Not a specific passion. Not some great enthusiasm for a certain subject but an undifferentiated passion that is there when we rise and is still with us when we retire at night.

A passion for life itself.

Anyone can have it. One need not be a member of Mensa or a graduate of Juilliard or the schools that train people in the arts. Nor is the eventual expression of that passion important. Once passion is there, the way a person does a thing becomes much more important than what is being done.

Passion itself it not enough. We are also, as Brando says, our experience. The expression of this passion will be limited to this storage-and-retrieval system in our conscious and subconscious minds. It is imperative, therefore, that we learn to see the good in everything that happens. We are our experiences. We are also in an even more important way our interpretation of those experiences.

There are no bad experiences, if you have a sense of humor. If you can see through to the actual meaning and import of an event. Humor acknowledges no logic. Humor knows that life is a problem which admits of no solution.

Nevertheless, we must act as if one did exist. We take this reality, interpose our peculiar genius, and produce our own art. My art is running. It is also writing these essays. But primarily it is the making of my character. I am creating the person I am, just as surely as Marlon Brando creates a person on the stage or in a film.

A good friend wrote me about a seventy-year-old named Lou who was once a professional ballroom dancer. Lou runs all day in a park in Miami trying to become his ideal physical self. Running is Lou's answer to the ever-present opposites of life and death. He is building himself a character, the invisible and permanent profile or marking of himself which can never die.

Chapter Twenty-three
On
Competing

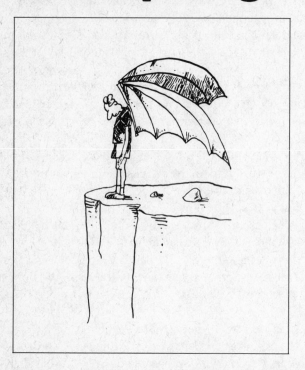

"... human nature abhors equilibrium. There is nothing more boring than ease and routine. We cannot stand for long the slow succession of uneventful days. We are never quite content with the status quo. It is nature that aims to achieve stability, nature that constantly seeks homeostasis. But human beings will not let things rest. We must be in motion."

Five minutes before the Fourth of July 10-Kilometer Pepsi Challenge Race the loudspeakers began to pour out "Rocky's Theme." There was a noticeable increase in movement on the plaza of the George Washington Bridge. Thousands of runners began walking and jogging to the starting line. The race was only moments away. The next half-hour for some, an hour for others, would be what the Greeks called the *agon*, the struggle. Johan Huizinga in his book *Homo Ludens* described it as play. We runners know better. We call it sport.

"The occasion," said Huizinga, "is sacred or festive." Today it was both. We were celebrating a secular feast. It was a day of holiday and history. A day that said all men were equal and all men were free. And we were putting the seal on it by freely taking an oath on the race that was to follow. Giving our word of honor to do our best.

There was a brief silence. Then the anthem. And now we were ready for what was to come. "It is an activity," Huizinga went on, "which proceeds within certain limits of time and place, in a visible order according to rules freely accepted and outside the sphere of necessity and material utility."

We were to proceed for 10 kilometers (about 6¼ miles) over the bridge into Manhattan and end up at Baker Field, an athletic facility of Columbia University. We knew the rules and accepted them. Runners are a law-abiding lot. But in the race we accept rules that are generally unenforceable. Cheating is not merely unethical, it is unintelligible. It destroys both the runner and the race.

One reason for this obedience is time. Time matters as much as space. Indeed, the real enemy is the digital clock at the finish line. That clock is the closure, the end, the judgment. And it has, as you can see, no relation to necessity or utility.

In those last moments I can feel the electricity in the crowd. There is a continual stirring. An excitement that leaps from one runner to another. "The mood," wrote Huizinga, "is one of rapture and enthusiasm." I feel that mood fill me. "Enthusiasm" is a strong word for strong feelings. I have them. Passion and daring and commitment to what is ahead. And rapture. I am seized by the whole event. The rest of the world falls away. Up until now I have felt reluctant to suffer, but now that is set aside. I cannot wait for that suffering to get underway.

The gun sounds, and we stream down an incline and spill out onto the bridge. The Hudson is on either side and in front Manhattan and the entire span empty of everything except runners. I am running the first mile too fast as I always do. I am filled with the exultation that Huizinga said accompanied the action. I am carried away by the race and the day and those around me. I feel larger than life and capable of anything.

A brief six minutes and the feeling is over. From now on another emotion identified by Huizinga will dominate—tension. Uncertainty about myself and the outcome will fill the rest of the race. I am in control, yet I am not in control. What will I face and will I be able to face it? I'll be running with that question from here to the end.

We come off the bridge and run upriver past The Cloisters. The going is fairly easy until a steep half-mile hill leading to the toll booths on the Henry Hudson Bridge, the turnaround point. That hill is my moment of truth. I am paying for the fast pace on the first mile. I hold nothing back, but my pace gets slower and slower. People are passing me, and my thighs can take no more pain. This is the race right here.

The top finally comes and then the long merciful downhill. Now I am passing those who passed me going up. I am feeling better than at any other time since the start. The race, I suddenly realize, is mine.

And that was the way it was through the finish. The digital clock read 38:38, my best time of the year. Others had done personal bests also. Baker Field was filled with happy runners in groups talking about the race and how it had been run. All around me it was as Huizinga described it. "Mirth and relaxation follow," he said.

Eventually we went to a small Irish bar a block or so away and sat drinking beer and telling each other what wonderful people we were. Not, of course, in words but with our eyes and our gestures and that bearing that comes with running the best you can on the Fourth of July.

I HAD DISCOVERED what every runner looks for. A race with a small field, a flat course and trophies in my age group. It was a Sunday event in a little seacoast town with less than 200 entrants and only a handful in the fifty-and-over group.

Then I saw him. He was already waiting at the starting line stripped to the waist, wearing a digital stopwatch and the telltale 500 number. He was lean and muscular and built for endurance. And not a gray hair on his head. I had found a race and gotten myself a tiger.

I knew then it would be no different from every other Sunday. The stage was set for the usual drama. Age-group racing does that. The confrontation with runners my own age makes every race a race within a race, a play within a play. Every race is a stage, and I become one of the actors.

The race is always a race against the clock. It is also a race for the best place in the multitude that faces the starter's gun. But when there is a prize for people of my vintage the race becomes pure Elizabethan drama.

In Greek drama it is man against the superhuman. The tragedy results when the hero or heroine sins against the gods. Our current theater is man against the world. The individual interests against the common good. The question is, Which is the stronger, the one standing alone or the one who gives to others? But the Elizabethan drama is man against himself. The plot unfolds and is determined by the flaws and faults of the protagonist. The ambition of Macbeth, the irresoluteness of Hamlet, the jealousy of Othello, make the play.

In the next 30 minutes or so this bare-chested, well-trained competent fifty-year-old runner was going to test me. He was going to search out the flaws in my character. He and I were about to produce, write and act out our own drama. It would be, as George Santayana wrote of athletics, a physical drama, in which all moral and emotional interests are involved. "The soul is stirred," he said, "in this spectacle that represents the basis of its whole life."

You might wonder why at my age I do these things. I could

easily have been at the beach or sitting over a late breakfast reading *The New York Times*. I could have been enjoying this summer Sunday like millions of others in this land. But no, here I am with but moments to the start, tying my shoes for the third time, taking the last ounces of my cola, exchanging greetings with those around me.

I have left behind the self and the equilibrium I have established over the years. I have come to the uncertainty and tension and the possibility of disaster that this race represents. I have put myself in a most difficult and trying situation when I could be peaceful and content at home.

Why do I feel this compulsion? Mainly, I believe, because human nature abhors equilibrium. There is nothing more boring than ease and routine. We cannot stand for long the slow succession of uneventful days. We are never quite content with the status quo. It is nature that aims to achieve stability, nature that constantly seeks homeostasis. But human beings will not let things rest. We must be in motion.

So I take this hard-won equilibrium, this self that I have made, and then establish a vacuum of deeds not yet done, achievements not yet mine. I say nay to all that has gone before, and I come to the race. I impose another test, another trial, another challenge to be experienced before I can claim to be me.

The playwrights know this sequence well. The equilibrium is first destroyed. Then there are moves and countermoves. There is the clash of wills. The issue is joined. The inevitable then occurs. The flaws of the individual are revealed. And they determine the outcome.

When the equilibrium is restored, what must be done has been done. The play comes full circle revealing what has always been potential in the situation and the people in it. Replay the drama and it comes out the same. Rerun the race and it does also. Only the growth and development of the characters can change it.

There were by now only seconds to go. I stood just behind my rival waiting for the curtain to go up on our private struggle. The gun went off. The play had begun.

WHEN THE GUN SOUNDED we went off as if tied together. Two fifty-and-over runners oblivious of the rest of the field. What was now of importance in this six-mile race in a little seacoast town would occur between us. The moves and countermoves, the clash of wills which would mark this drama, would be our moves and countermoves, and our personal clash of wills. The exposition, the confrontation, the climax and the denouement would all occur in the less than five yards that would separate us for the entire race. And the new equilibrium we would find at the finish line would come from who we truly were.

The race does what every good drama does. It tells the truth. Each move, each event, is an actual happening. And everything that happens has an effect on everything else. In race as in drama there is no unimportant information. From gun to finish line my every action would reveal the inner man who prompted it.

The stranger who was my opponent and rival would also be colleague and friend. Together we would write and act out this drama. Together we would explore this new experience. Together we would gain a new appreciation of ourselves. Together we would make this struggle an image of our inner struggle to make sense out of our lives.

We went through the first mile in six minutes. The exposition was already taking place. His best pace was my best pace. The issue was now joined. He made the next move. A slight acceleration in pace. He was using the classical strategy in the confrontation between my speed and his endurance. He was trying to break away from me or at the least take the sting out of my kick at the finish.

My tactic was simple. Sit in behind. Let him do the work. Take him at the end. His had become equally simple. Increase the pace until I let him go. The pressure of this speed eventually became unbearable, so I took the lead in an attempt to slow it down. He would have none of that and immediately went out in front once more.

And so went those first few miles. It had become a matter of the body and the will. Emotion can help, but reason is useless. After the first rush the race is a matter of character and talent. One runner rarely out-thinks another. The runner knows what must be done and then musters the courage to do it.

He knew his role; I knew mine. His, a continued striving to leave me behind. Mine, a persistent refusal to allow that to happen. So on I went, the arms getting heavy, the chest desperate for air, the legs now filling with pain. He was calling on his body for even more effort, and I attached to his right shoulder and was paying the price.

This was the perennial struggle between human wills and within individual human wills now seen plain. We had gone through the exposition and the confrontation. Now we were in the last mile. He still led with me a step behind. Neither of us would give an inch. We matched stride for stride. I was running on virtues and values I never knew I had. I just would not give up. Nor would he.

I was now no longer merely racing against him. I was racing against me at my best. That was what he had come to represent. He was my alter ego. The best possible me. And only my best effort would beat him. He was in a similar predicament. He had not been able to shake me. I was still there off his right shoulder as I had been almost from the beginning. It was a signal to do more or less.

We made a turn then, and far down the road I could see the banner over the finish line. My friend mustered his final challenge. His pace went up a notch or two. Mine did also. And we came down that last stretch head to head, chest to chest, like a team of matched horses.

By now he was flat out and so was I. With less than a hundred yards to go we were still neck and neck. When I thought of that later I realized we had both won. We had done what had been asked of us and surpassed ourselves in the doing. This tense struggle of wills and bodies had told us truly who we were.

What happened after that was anticlimactic. With 50 yards to go I pulled the trigger and surged forward. I was running on muscle fibers I had not used and he did not have. Pain and exhaustion and shortness of breath were no longer deterrents. He was no match for this madness. So I won the 50-and-over.

I had beaten him but it really didn't matter. Seconds later we were shaking hands and congratulating each other. We stood there happy and content and more than a little proud. We had made the theoretical fact that we were born to be heroes a reality.

Chapter Twenty-four
On Rewarding

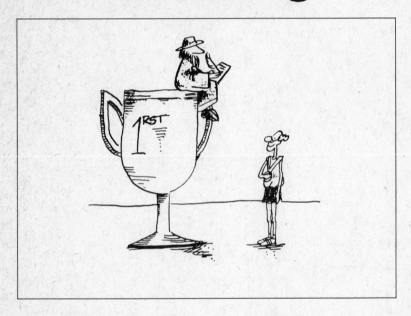

"The trophy announces the completeness of
the event. It is the final act that isolates,
encloses and memorializes the race just run.
It need not be something you can see or feel
or place on your mantel. . . . But there
should be *something* that makes the contest
a matter of record."

THE NEXT DAY, people kept asking me how I had done. At first, I answered that I didn't finish. Then I began saying that I *couldn't* finish. What I should have said was, "I hit the wall." I should have told them right off that I hit it. Then they might have understood.

In any case, that is what happened. In this 1980 Boston Marathon, I finally hit the wall. After years of reading about it, hearing about it, lecturing about it, I had totally and irrevocably hit the wall. After seventeen years of successful Bostons, I failed to finish. I reached the Prudential in a trolley, not on foot.

Just past the 21-mile mark, coming down the hill at Boston College, I knew I was finished. There had been, however, a hint of disaster all day. I had come to Boston on the strength of my best-ever marathon and was attempting to duplicate it—a dangerous thing to do at any time but particularly with the temperature in the 70s. There was a cloudless sky, so the sun was contributing another 10 to 20 degrees. The following wind virtually eliminated heat dissipation by air conduction.

On such a day, initial pace is of paramount importance. When there is excessive heat stress, speed increases dehydration, elevates body temperature, and, of prime importance, rapidly uses up the muscle-glycogen stores. On such a day, I should have been thinking of running 30 seconds a mile slower than my usual time. Instead I was thinking of running 30 seconds a mile *faster*. I had always prided myself on prudence in such circumstances, but like many other runners I was already thinking about qualifying for next year. Instead of running according to our bodies, we ran against the clock. It was the most competitive Boston Marathon I ever ran.

At around the 15-mile mark in Newton Lower Falls, I began to feel uneasy about the outcome. The long downhill there was much more difficult than in other years. Then, on the upgrade, I discovered I was losing the drive in my legs. There was no bounce. I had no lift. I could hear my footstrike, a sure sign of losing form and coordination. I was like a pitcher who had found there was no steam on his fastball. I was in trouble.

Nonetheless, I negotiated the Newton hills and got past Heartbreak without too much additional difficulty. It was on the long descent past the crowds at Boston College that I began to come apart. My pace slowed until I was running in slow motion. My arms were moving more than my legs. All the way to the foot of the hill, I ran—rather, moved in a grotesque caricature of running—all the while hoping that I would be all right once I got on the flat and could run again.

Going downhill at that point is always bad. The front thigh muscles always protest. Each step becomes extremely painful. I had gone through that before and then recovered to run well to the finish, so I hoped that would happen again when I finally reached the bottom.

"Now," I said to myself, "it will be better." But it wasn't. If anything, it was worse. The pain was still there, and now an overwhelming weariness. The muscles had become lifeless. They had lost not only power and coordination but shock-absorption as well. Every step not only hurt my thighs but was doing terrible things to my knees.

Nevertheless, I persisted. With each step my pace became slower, but I refused to walk. There was simply no question of walking. No matter what happens, I told myself, I will not walk. I had never walked in Boston, and there would be no first time.

I could hear the crowd encouraging me. Some called out, "Looking good." Others yelled, "You can make it." The more perceptive shouted, "Tough it out," and "Hang in there." Now and then, I would hear what seemed to be the rallying cry for this year's run, "Go for it."

It was going for it that had gotten me into this state. Had I run prudently during the first half, I would now be taking it in, running my body and heart out but finishing. Now I was reduced to this private little hell, my eyes fixed on my shadow in front of me, watching this pantomime. I was apparently running but actually not. I was moving up and down, but not forward. I was virtually running in place. And all the while, I was losing any sense of the crowd and the race and where I was. My life became that one thought: keep running.

Then I felt a hand and looked up. There was a friend beside me. She was watching the race and seeing me in this state, she had rushed out.

"Don't you want to walk, George?" she asked. She was a mother talking to a child. By now she had her arm around me, holding me up. I was still running, and there she was standing there holding me up. I was no longer moving forward, but I was not going to walk.

"George, don't you want to walk?" she asked again. She had come out of the crowd to save me from myself. I looked at her standing there, her face full of sympathy and care and love. I knew it was the end.

"Nina," I said, "all I want is someone to take me home."

Then a trolley appeared as if she had summoned it, and she got me on it. When I boarded it, the twenty or so people inside sent up a cheer. That upset me at first.

"Why cheer me?" I asked them. "I didn't even finish."

It apparently didn't matter. Someone came up and offered me orange juice, and someone else gave me his seat. So I rode to the Prudential, beginning to feel good about the whole thing.

The wall, I thought, can be a peak experience.

THE AWARDS CEREMONY was drawing to a close. My partner, Althea, and I were standing just below the officials' box, pressed against the rope controlling the crowd. Peter Roth of the New York Road Runners Club was about to announce the winners of the 120-and-over division of the Trevira Twosome.

The Trevira was then only in its second year, but it had already caught the imagination of runners. Pairing male and female runners, and grouping them according to aggregate age, adds interest and enthusiasm for everyone in the race. Some runners even bypass the Boston Marathon to run the Trevira a week later. The field totals more than 3,000.

I had sought Althea out after seeing her run a fine 10-kilometer in Bermuda and come back the following day with a respectable marathon. Most important, she was 63; we had become the team to beat in our age group. Now we were waiting to see if we had done it.

We must have won, I thought. It had been a tough race. Running 10 miles only a week after Boston had to be tough. I had been walking downstairs backward until two days earlier, but in this race the old moves had come back. My time had been good, too. I had shaved my pre-race estimate of 64 minutes by a few seconds.

Then it had been a matter of waiting for Althea. She had predicted a time of 1:18, and I knew I could set my watch on that. Althea runs like a metronome. A few seconds past 1:18 on the digital clock, I saw her enter the chute. She is a little over medium height, quite thin, with straight gray hair and features that remind me of Amelia Earhart. That moment, Althea looked like a very competent runner.

The ceremonies began more than an hour later. By that time, most of the thousands of runners and spectators had departed. But several hundred waited in the rain for the awards. Here and there were umbrellas, and most of the winners sought refuge under an awning suspended from the Road Runners' van.

Applause went up for the overall winners: Herb Lindsay and Margaret Groos. Both had set American road records for 10 miles. They had beaten the team of Frank Shorter and Joan Benoit. Althea and I were in distinguished company.

More categories were announced. The various winners went up to receive boxes containing huge silver bowls and then departed, taking their friends with them. The rain continued to fall intermittently. The skies gradually became darker. Officials began taking down the finishing chute. The starting-line banner went next. Then the other banners disappeared.

During a lull, a man who appeared to be my age asked what our team's elapsed time had been. I told him.

"We beat you," he said. "I ran 67 minutes, and my wife ran 72."

All that waiting, I thought, and we were only runners-up.

The computer had to dig deep to get winners in the higher age-groups. Peter Roth apologized for the delay. More people left. Then he called out the 100-and-over winner—the husband-and-wife team. I had worried needlessly. I had forgotten to ask how old he was. Althea and I were sure winners in the 120-plus group.

By now there was no one left but Althea and me, her husband and three friends waiting to take me for a beer. There was no evidence left of the run. Central Park Drive was empty. Even the officials' box was empty. Peter Roth had gone to the van to get the final results.

Then the door of the van opened and Peter came out, paper in hand. He strode to the stand, mounted it and faced the nonexistent crowd.

"I want you to hold it down," he shouted. Then he proceeded as if all 3,000 runners were there. He raised his hand, gesturing for order.

"Further," he said, "there will be no storming this stand to congratulate the winners. I'm sure they can give you time afterward. In the 120-and-over category, from Huntington Station, Long Island, Althea Wetherbee, and her partner, from Red Bank, New Jersey, George Sheehan. Their elapsed time: 2 hours, 22 minutes and 2 seconds."

Althea and I climbed onto the box and faced out, seeing the faces of people we had run with, reliving the joy we had felt crossing the finish line—and feeling, too, joy in this marvelous charade.

Peter asked us to say a few words to the multitude, which we did, and then finally he gave us our boxes. They were empty. It was the final twist. Both Althea and I broke up. Everyone was laughing as if laughter had just been discovered.

When we made our way down the steps, two officials who had stayed through the whole ceremony came over. They were wearing Trevira sweatshirts. One took his off and give it to Althea, and the other took his off and gave it to me. Then he went into the van, came out with two New York Marathon slickers, and gave one to each of us. The winners of the 120-and-over division of the Trevira Twosome departed in style, the cheers of the crowd ringing in our ears.

THESE MORNINGS, I drink my let's-start-the-day coffee from a mug with sea gulls painted on it. It is the most cherished memento I ever won in a race. The house is filled with medals and plaques and prizes from other races, but I rarely look at them. The mug is there every morning to remind me that I am a runner.

I won that mug in a 5-mile race in Spring Lake, New Jersey. There were 1,500 runners in the race, with the first 140 finishers receiving mugs. Without age groups or special divisions to differentiate men from women, the starter fired his gun and the first 140 runners back got mugs. No race could be simpler.

I do not recall a more competitive race. Spring Lake is a coastal town, a resort where every square foot is at sea level. There isn't a hill to be seen. No matter how a course is laid out in Spring Lake, it's going to be as flat as a billiard table.

You would think the absence of hills would have made the race easier. Not so. Hills make it easier to forget the runners in front of you. Hills turn your thoughts to survival; finishing becomes more important than where you finish. A flat course has no such distractions. You are compelled to maintain contact with the leaders for as long as you can. And at Spring Lake this desire was intensified. No one was giving up. No one would let anyone else pass. It was every racer for himself.

We went out, 1,500 strong, at flank speed, trusting that we could hold on to a pace that was too fast for most of us yet commonly arrived at. I heard my split at the end of the first mile: 5:42—my fastest mile of the year, and yet there seemed to be hundreds of runners ahead of me.

After the first blistering mile, it was time to hang on, never give up, pick off a runner now and then, but mostly not to let anyone pass me. And no one did until the 4-mile mark. He was half my age and probably double my strength. But I stayed on his heels, fighting the pain and the weariness through those interminable final minutes. I was even able to sprint the last 50 yards and storm through the finish line, where the officials handed out placement cards. I looked down and read mine: 136. The mug was mine.

Why did I need a coffee-mug trophy? After all, I had the Spring Lake T-shirt and race number to keep. Weren't they sufficient souvenirs of that day? Why another memento of that occasion? I'm not sure myself. I often leave a race without picking up my award. The shirt, the number, the companionship and the competition are memories enough. Yet many sports are synonymous with the prize: hockey and the Stanley Cup, college football and the Heisman, golf and the Masters green coat, yachting and America's Cup. The word "prize" comes from the same Latin root as "price" and "praise." The prize reflects the price the athlete paid for the victory, and the praise from spectators and fellow contestants.

The mug proves I am an athlete. The word "athlete" comes from the root word *aethlon*, which also means prize. The seemingly inconsequential coffee mug is proof of my new existence as a runner. It is evidence of the contest—a contest that is different from a game. It is not fun or pleasurable. The Greeks called such a struggle *agon*, from which we get the word "agony." I have gone through that agony, I have done my best, and now I have the trophy to prove it.

The trophy announces the completeness of the event. It is the final act that isolates, encloses and memorializes the race just run. It need not be something you can see or feel or place on your mantel; it may simply be raising the victor's hand. But there should be *something* that makes the contest a matter of record.

The trophy also acts as a sacrament. It is an outward sign of an inward happening. The trophy asserts that human beings are willing to push themselves to the limit simply to prove they can do it. The prize, the race and human limitations are inextricably tied together in the mystery that is sport. The explanation, therefore, remains unexplainable. There is no logic in illogical acts.

There was also no logic or explanation for the way I acted when I picked up my mug at the officials' table. Holding it aloft to look at it, I savored the feel of the handle under my fingers. Carrying it proudly so all could see, I jogged back to my gear—a victory jog instead of the usual exhausted walk. The mug had become the seal on an event I would never forget.

When I drink my coffee from the "trophy," I remember that race. And there is even more in that memory than the actual happening, more than placing 136th and the good feeling afterward. My mug helps me start the day, ready for whatever comes. Because of that race and other races now almost lost in memory, I know I am good and whole and holy; that what I must do I *can* do, and that the world is filled with people ready to work and suffer and enjoy with me.

The real trophy, you see, is not the coffee mug at all. It is the person drinking from it. My real trophy is the self that running and racing have made me.

Chapter Twenty-five
On
Sharing

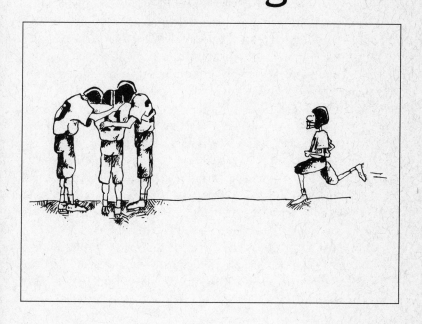

"What we are doing is past analyzing. I know only that I cannot lose my attachment to my companions. If I do, I will become once more a frail individual attempting a task that is at once irrational and unnecessary."

WHEN WE LINED UP for the race, the field was at least one-third black, another third Hispanic. Not the usual entry for a road race, but then the El Barrio 10-Kilometer in Spanish Harlem was not the usual road race.

I was there because there was no race that Sunday in Central Park, none on the seacoast where I live. I had no choice but to enter what seemed to me to be occupied territory. I had set out for Third Avenue and 100th Street with some apprehension. I was worried about my car and my belongings, if not my person.

I am as prejudiced as any American. We live in a melting pot that has never quite melted. Most of our brotherhood is symbolic, not concrete. We avoid situations that would force us to act upon our beliefs. We are all for brotherhood, but we stay clear of our brothers.

This is in some ways normal. Humanity, says Erik Erikson, is inherently inclined to differentiate itself into various sub-species: race, class, nation, etc. The resultant allegiances, he points out, bring out the best in man in terms of loyalty, self-sacrifice and charity. They also, however, bring out the worst. Outsiders become threats to our basic needs of survival and security, of acceptance and self-esteem. They become expendable.

Prejudice is an adult disease. Nevertheless, its incubation begins in childhood. It doesn't take very long for a child to be taught that other people are different. It doesn't take very many years to establish strata of acceptability. When that happens, childhood is lost.

When I was a kid in Brooklyn, we stayed in our own section. We learned that where there were differences in race and language and ethnic background, there were tensions and even dangers. We knew enough to stay out of what we called "tough neighborhoods." We came to see strangers as threats to ourselves and our property.

Because I still retain the vestiges of that boy growing up in Brooklyn, those feelings—some conscious, some subconscious— were present when I parked my car a block or so away from the starting line in Spanish Harlem.

Third Avenue was already alive with runners and families with children of all sizes. The playground at the intersection was filled with people getting their numbers and officials giving directions. There were tables of T-shirts and entry blanks for future races, and on the side paraphernalia for the party that would follow the race. In the background flowed music with an insistent, catchy beat. The usual movement and excitement and enthusiasm before a race were intensified.

By the time we began that slow walk to the starting line, I felt completely at home. This was the same as any other race on any other Sunday. Ahead of me lay the familiar 6.2 miles that would test my tolerance of pain, my capacity for suffering, the limits of my will, the extent of my tenacity. And as usual, I was about to undergo this trial in community with others, themselves engaged in the same enterprise. I was once more just a runner among runners.

The gun sounded, and within a few strides we were neither black nor white, Irish nor Hispanic. We were simply a homogeneous horde of panting runners. At the mile mark, all I could see around me were fellow sufferers. Pain knows no color; exhaustion has no creed. The language of the body is universal; it speaks to all in the same way.

The race disdains distinctions. Fatigue and discomfort and shortness of breath make us all brothers. They purge us of the fear and the hate and the pride that breed prejudice. The race cleanses us, using a pace we can barely sustain, for a distance we can barely traverse and a length of time that is at the outer limit of our physical ability. We are renewed by being totally spent.

After I finished, I moved with the others through the cheering crowd into the playground, where the party had already begun. I was met there with soda and beer, beans and barbecued chicken. All around were music and laughter and a great good feeling.

You see, there are things that unify us. There are emotions that demonstrate clearly our essential oneness. These experiences bring us, no matter how diverse the expression of our humanity, into an acceptance and trust and belief in each other.

One of them is pain; we had that in the race. Another is sport; we had that in the race, too. Finally, there is celebration, and I have attended few better parties than the one we had after the race in Spanish Harlem.

The awards ceremony came last. There was applause for everyone, and just a little more for those runners who had names like Hector and Carlos and Jose. The 50-and-over trophy went to an Irishman from a suburb in New Jersey. He told the crowd he had been born two blocks from here and had grown up in Harlem.

"I want to thank the people of *el barrio*," he said, "for an outstanding day in my life."

As we used to say in Brooklyn, that goes double for me.

TWO DECADES AGO, no one influential in running or exercise physiology or physical education had any idea that women could run long distances, much less marathons. Women were restricted to the sprints.

"I had wanted to run 20 years ago," I was told by a thirty-nine-year-old woman about to start a Boston Marathon. "But I wasn't allowed to. They thought women were too delicate. We were not permitted to run over 220 yards."

History, however, has proven that women are capable of running a marathon. It is now evident that whatever a man can do in distance running, a woman can also do. As the number of women long-distance runners increases, they present continuing proof that women respond to training the same ways as men. They make the most of what they were given at birth.

When a woman becomes a runner, she develops her own level of competence. Each one is able to establish herself somewhere on that long continuum of men and women who compete together. When I race, there are women ahead of me, women behind me. I see them only as fellow runners. They train as I train. In the race, they make the same effort, feel the same pain, suffer just as much in that drive toward the finish. And afterward they share the same pleasant exhaustion, the same satisfaction. Running and the race have made us, male and female, one.

A woman told me about this new attitude she had discovered in running. "For the first time in my life," she said, "I am considered as another human being rather than a woman doing fairly well at a man's job."

One reason this occurs is that the woman runner feels this way about *herself*. Once a woman thinks she is capable, she is. Once a woman discounts the difference between the male and female athlete, it ceases to exist.

Plato thought much the same way. In *The Republic*, he stated, "Women should take part in all the same occupations as men, both in peace and in war, acting as guardians and hunting with the men like hounds."

Women, he said, should be treated the same as men—both mentally and physically—and trained in identical skills.

William James joined in this plea for the full development of physical potential. In his *Gospel of Relaxation*, he referred to the social and educational changes in Norwegian women once they had taken to skiing.

"I hope," James wrote, "that here in America, more and more the ideal of the well-trained and vigorous body will be maintained neck-and-neck as the two coequal halves of the higher education for men and women alike."

Women now know that they have the same enormous endurance capabilities that men have. Once an achievement is seen as possible, it will be achieved. Once a woman believes she can run a marathon, she will run it.

The Establishment is always a step behind these developments. The exercise physiologists, those professors in human performance, are just now agreeing that women are indeed capable of running respectable marathons. The American College of Sports Medicine recently published an opinion paper by experts on this issue. It presents all the current evidence and gives this final opinion:

"There exists no conclusive scientific or medical evidence that long-distance running is contra-indicated for the healthy, trained female athlete. . . . The ACSM recommends that females be allowed to compete at the same distances in which their male counterparts compete."

This is, of course, old news to Plato and James, and to thousands of women marathoners. It will, nevertheless, do some good if it enlightens those educators and coaches and physicians whose present policy is to restrict rather than expand women's participation in sports.

I AM STANDING, waiting for the gun, at a 10-kilometer race in Central Park. On a cold, wet day that normally would deter me from leaving the house, I wait impatiently to attack the 6.2 miles of challenging terrain that lie ahead of me. There are 4,500 runners in this race. The starting line has become a crush of bodies. I am pressed in on all sides. No longer the solitary runner, I have become a member of a mob—one of a crowd.

Whenever I race, I take on the characteristics described by the French psychologist Gustave LeBon in his classic treatise *The Crowd: A Study of the Popular Mind*. When a certain number of individuals gather in a crowd for the purpose of action, he said, there result certain new psychological qualities.

"Visible social phenomena appear to be the result of an immense unconscious working that is a rule beyond our analysis," LeBon wrote.

The race is just such an unexplainable, visible social phenomenon. People can see some practical reasons for running but almost none for racing. That is because what lies ahead is not an intellectual act; it is an emotional event.

Crowds never accomplish deeds demanding any degree of intelligence. Crowds have to do with the unconscious—with instincts, passions and emotions common to all. On the starting line, we are all equal. We may differ markedly in intellect and mental ability—but not in character, not in the capabilities of our unconscious. The starting line is where all these psychological events occur. It is here that each runner becomes part of this new being, the collective "us" about to run this race.

As I stand here, I already possess some of the qualities enumerated by LeBon. The first is the sentiment of invincible power. In this pushing together of bodies, the task before me no longer appears formidable. I draw strength from those about me. Their good cheer, their indifference to the ordeal now only minutes away, fills me with the same overwhelming confidence. I know that my powers are equal to whatever is to come.

The gun sounds. As a horde, we stream down the first hill, then up the next at almost breakneck speed. All of us are caught in the contagion that seizes groups. Reason departs, instinct takes over.

"In a crowd," wrote LeBon, "man descends several rungs in the developmental ladder. Isolated, he may be a cultivated individual. In a crowd, he is a barbarian—that is, a creature acting by instinct."

The first mile is all of this. I am drawn along by the contagion, kept at this speed by my new suggestibility. I believe that this incredible pace is not only necessary but possible, and I hold it —or at least try. But try as I may, I lose some ground. The army that started is beginning to break down into platoons.

It is from this point that the race becomes a transforming experience. The race is an instance of a crowd that has a positive effect on those in it. Too often, we think of crowds as bad or criminal. But a crowd can also be heroic. Great actions, LeBon pointed out, are rarely performed in cold blood.

This race I am in may not be a great action, but what is left after that first mile can only be called heroic. Pain and persistence are now our common experience. We have a common mind which has become a common reflex.

We have focused down to the running of this race. It has become the most important thing we will ever do. Everything else is blotted out of our minds.

"Crowds," wrote LeBon, "are cognizant only of simple and extreme sentiments." We know that. We have no doubt or uncertainty about the extreme importance of what we are doing.

William Barrett, the philosopher, has written about this feeling: "The runner does not doubt the race as long as he continues to strain every nerve and muscle in the effort. If he eases up for a moment, he is likely to see the whole thing for what it is: an absurd and useless display, not worth the effort."

This almost never occurs, Barrett admitted. Writing about the last finisher in the Boston Marathon, he called him an image of the man of faith: "There simply cannot be a question of his quitting."

For me, this "absurd and useless display" is taking on more meaning. For me and those in my platoon, there is no question of quitting. We find strength where there is no strength left. Pain becomes bearable, because everyone else is bearing it. And inside of that pain, we find energies that only agony will release.

We are now moving into areas behind logic and reason. What we are doing is past analyzing. I know only that I cannot lose my attachment to my companions. If I do, I will become once more a frail individual attempting a task that is at once irrational and unnecessary.

I do not allow that to happen. Alone on this day, I would long since have given up. I can do what I am doing only when I am one of this crowd—because I am a racer with my fellow racers.

"Take me in," I say—sometimes aloud, sometimes under my breath, sometimes as a plea, sometimes as a prayer. And they do. They always do.

"DID ANYTHING MEMORABLE occur during the race?" The questioner at the other end of the telephone was in a Charleston radio station. I was standing in a phone booth wearing borrowed sweats and holding the sixty-and-over trophy for the Cooper River Bridge 10-Kilometer Race. Outside I could see the remnants of the 2,000-entry field still enjoying themselves and their refreshments.

I searched my mind for something a news reporter would think memorable. Someone hit by a car, or collapsing from the effort. What man had bitten a dog during the race? What incident that would interest those people who spend their days listening to what happens to other people?

The man was patient. He repeated the question. I remained silent. I was still thinking. I did not tell him about the day before. I had been picked up at the airport by a stranger who was also a runner. This morning I was taken to the race by this same man, now a close friend. I had spent less than 12 hours in a strange house I now and forever would regard as another home. I was as comfortable in Charleston as I was in my old running shoes.

I did not tell him about sitting in the car at the starting line. It was too cold this blustery day to warm up. The flags on the *Yorktown*, berthed at the Point, were straight out and flapping. When the race began the first mile was straight into that driving wind, yet the huge mass of runners made it like being in the eye of a hurricane. There was practically no air movement at all.

I did not tell him about the bridge. It loomed up just after we made the hairpin turn at the mile mark. From then on the wind would be at our backs. Never a real hindrance, it became a help. It pushed us toward this narrow ribbon of steel rising into the sky like something in a fairy story.

I have run other bridges—the George Washington, the Golden Gate, the Verrazano. All give the impression of solidity and function. For all their architectural brilliance, those bridges are matter-of-fact utilitarian structures. They are simply there to carry things to the other side.

Not so the Cooper River Bridge. It is a thin double span that crosses two rivers and goes for some two and a half miles to a destination that must be accepted on faith. This bridge carried us up and over and through to some distant land, to a mythical Charleston. It was not a bridge, it was an adventure.

Nor did I tell him about the woman runner. She appeared beside me on the first rise. Her pace was steady, relentless and unforgiving. I knew she would not vary one iota from that stride and speed until the finish line. I gave her the reins and concentrated on just staying with her.

We went together, scudding down the other side and up the second rise, finally spilling out into East Bay Street in Charleston. If there ever was Heaven in a race, this was it. I had shed my hat and gloves and thrown my shirt over my head so I was running bare-chested in this perfect weather. The wind was at my back, the course flat, and I still felt fresh.

Then came the turning into Queen Street, and everyone began to pick up the pace. "How far to go?" gasped a lanky teenager beside me. "A half mile," I said. He took off like a colt who has seen its mother. His tow-head disappeared in the crowd up front.

Then I heard, "On your left . . . ," and his place was taken by two runners, George Halman, who is blind, and a companion who was joined to him by a cord at the wrists. Until I saw George I thought I was doing my absolute best. Now I was spurred to do more. I went with him hoping to share in his strength and courage. I drew up to his shoulder and drew on his guts and determination.

We went that way to the end. The digital clock read 39:05, my best this year. Afterward, I stood at the chute for a long time congratulating those who finished behind me, seeing in their happy and contented faces the happiness and contentment in mine. The feeling of being special filled those beautiful Charleston streets.

Then I joined a group of Irishmen surrounding a truck with a keg of beer. Later I wandered down to the ceremony at the Cistern and received my award. It was the perfect end of a perfect day.

The man was still waiting for an answer. "Did anything memorable occur during the race?" he asked once more.

"No," I said, "it was just like all those other races we run every weekend."

Chapter Twenty-six
On Striving

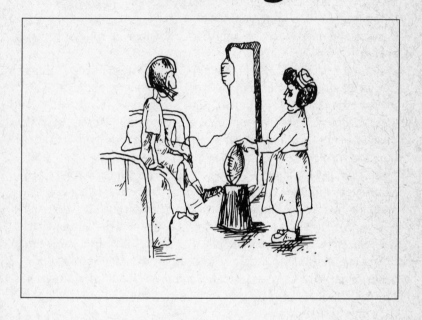

"Winning is never having to say I quit."

THERE ARE THINGS about myself I would rather not know. My IQ, for instance. I have no idea what it is and no intention of finding out. Either way, high or low, the news would be bad.

I would be distressed if my score was low, because I would rather not know my limitations. A low IQ could dissuade me from reaching for something within my grasp.

On the other hand, if it was high, I would be under the gun to produce more than ever before. There is nothing worse than being told you are quite capable of something that you know will stretch you to your very limit. There would no longer be any excuse for failure.

The IQ test identifies mental prodigies. A test of physical potential is equally disturbing. It identifies physical geniuses. This measurement might be called the "physical quotient," but instead it is known as the maximal oxygen uptake test. This test measures the system's capacity to transport oxygen from the lungs to the contracting muscles during exercise.

The major physiological changes that occur during fitness programs are usually measured in two ways: physical work capacity and maximal oxygen uptake. Work capacity is the ability to finish a distance. It has to do with endurance, not speed. This capacity may improve enormously, while there may be only a minor increase in oxygen uptake. Unless a person starting a fitness program is grossly overweight and completely out of shape, the oxygen uptake values usually do not increase more than 20 percent during training.

Oxygen uptake indicates the ability for all-out effort. In general, the maximal oxygen uptake determines where you will finish in a 5- or 10-mile race. With a high uptake, you'll finish up front. With a low uptake, you'll finish far back in the pack.

Although I have stuck to my decision not to learn my IQ score, I decided to have my oxygen uptake measured. It was a great mistake. It caused me as many problems as would have occurred with the disclosure of my IQ.

Knowing my oxygen uptake means that I now know exactly what times I should run in the mile, at 10 kilometers and in the marathon. I also know the absolute best times I can hope to achieve. This raises two problems: First, there is no excuse to do worse. Second, there is no hope to do better. What I can do is already programmed into my body. My responsibility is to get that performance out of it, fully realizing that achievements beyond are reserved for others more gifted than I.

I don't like living with this type of predestination. I no longer dream of doing better than my maximal oxygen uptake will let me. And I am no longer allowed to feel good about a race time that is just a mite slower than the one in the charts of my oxygen uptake.

Having this information seems to turn my body into a racing car that can do so much and no more, destined to live with my specific level of performance. A footrace seems to become a race between machines with different engine capacities.

Fortunately, winning is never this predetermined. For me, winning is a matter of doing my absolute best on a particular day. It is a matter of enduring pain, never relaxing when I feel good and maintaining contact as long as I can with the runners around me, even those better than I. Winning is never forgetting that I am running against the unforgiving clock—and not against the companions who race along with me. Winning is never having to say I quit.

So the war between my maximal oxygen uptake and me continues. In some races, I equal the predicted times. In others, I am far below them. Sometimes I am upset over the injustice of the fact that I am hurting as much as those who will finish minutes and even hours ahead of me. At other times, I am satisfied that the pain means I am getting the most possible out of this aging, finite body. When I translate the race into minutes and seconds, winning becomes a matter of breaking even. Winning is ending in a tie with my maximum performance potential.

I recall once holding a gasping conversation on this subject during a race in Central Park. One runner said he had a maximal oxygen uptake of 65 milliliters per kilogram per minute. My reading is 56.

"What does that mean?" he asked.

"It means," I said, "that you are dogging it back here with us. You should be a half mile ahead."

That is always my worry: dogging it, not getting the most out of what I have. That is my burden, and a terrible one it is. Every race imposes on me a duty not to cheat on myself, and in every race I must respond.

After an agonizing stretch run at the finish of a race in Van Cortlandt Park, an official came up to me and said, "George, you have guts."

I sat there wearily looking at him, and then said, "But why does it have to be that way in every race?"

Whether I know my IQ or not, my maximal oxygen uptake or not, there is no escaping the necessity to do my best, to fulfill my potential. Whether I am a success or a failure is recognized by every cell in my body.

THE FRIDAY NIGHT before the New York Marathon I spoke at a spaghetti dinner given by a local running club. Before the talk to the 100 runners and their families I loaded up on the bread and beer and pasta. And I shared in the excitement and enthusiasm and anticipation they all felt. Then in the question-and-answer period that followed someone asked me if I was going to run the marathon. Without hesitation I answered, "Yes."

Until that dinner I would have said "No." For the previous week I had thought of any number of legitimate reasons not to run. Primarily, I had not gotten in the necessary training. The current marathon pretraining programs prescribe a gradual buildup over three to six months to where the runner is doing at least 60 and preferably 70 miles a week. I have always run marathons on a good deal less. In fact I have never run 70 miles in one week and don't intend to. Two to three hours a week of easy running and a weekly race have been my premarathon routine over the years.

But this year my training had dipped far below even my minimum. Travel, colds and injuries had cut into my time on the roads. And when I was healthy I had raced so much I was too tired to train. My mileage in the last month was less than what most runners preparing for this race do in a week.

Then there were the calf cramps. In several recent races I had some ominous warnings in my calves. Cramps that were severe enough to slow me down on two occasions. Suppose I got a cramp (and it seemed like a distinct possibility) in some godforsaken spot in Brooklyn or the Bronx and I had to walk in.

Even if I was able to run without injury it would undoubtedly be in some undistinguished time. In coming months whenever the subject of the New York Marathon came up I would have to apologize for my time. I once ran the White Rock Marathon in Dallas after a long layoff in 3:28. Quite respectable under the circumstances. But few people let me explain the circumstances. So rather than be a bore, I just told them my time and let them think I was over the hill and going through an accelerated phase of degeneration.

I had this all in mind when I rose to speak that Friday night. I had even investigated the possibility of other races that day, a five-miler perhaps or some easy 10-kilometer run. But the closest event I could find was in Richmond, Virginia.

Then as I looked around me at those runners, I knew I had to be in it. One of the worst feelings in the world is that of missing something. The feeling that everything is going on somewhere else. Those people in front of me were what William James calls "the faithful fighters." And they were silently saying to me the words James used on the fainthearted who declined to go on, or the words of Henry IV when he greeted the tardy Crillon after a great victory: "Hang yourself, brave Crillon! We fought at Arques and you were not there."

That Friday night I knew I wanted to join in the fight. It was easier to risk pain and embarrassment and failure and the possibility of walking home from the Bronx than to miss this great and wonderful struggle.

So on Sunday I was there at Fort Wadsworth with 14,000 others, getting my number verified, fortifying myself with coffee and doughnuts and using the world's longest urinal. All my reluctance had gone. I was impatient to get underway.

The first twenty miles were a delight. You have heard of automatic writing that flows out of the writer from some unapprehended source. Those first twenty miles were automatic running.

Almost effortless, the 7-minute miles spun on and on. At 10 miles the digital clock read 1:10:10, and at 20 it was 2:20:10. An almost incredible consistency. Then I passed a sign that said, "Salazar 2:08:13, World Record." It was an inspiration. He had gone for it, so would I.

But from then on it was everything the last 6 miles of a marathon is said to be. Try as I might, my pace kept slowing. My form began to go. I lost the strength and flow that had marked the early going. Now the pain became a constant presence in my legs and thighs. And on the hills it filled my arms and chest.

I was constantly losing time to the clock. With a mile to go I was still uncertain about finishing. But those about me were still running so I assumed that I could and must. By now I was on Central Park South heading for Columbus Circle. The avenue has a slight upgrade with poor footing and was strangely devoid of spectators cheering the runners. I find this stretch always the most trying of the entire marathon. Here pain and exhaustion fuse with an intense desire just to give up. I want to say enough is enough. This whole enterprise is a mistake. It is too much for me.

But then I made the turn into the park and heard the cheering up ahead, and there they were, thousands of people lining the road and filling the grandstands and calling out my name. That was all I needed. I went up that last terrible hill to the finish line as if it didn't exist.

So hang yourself, dear reader, if we ran the New York Marathon and you were not there.

GOD WAS WATCHING. If there is any explanation for the 1982 Boston Marathon, that was it. The winner in collapse. Another finishing with a broken leg. A third crossing the line reciting her prayers. Thousands in various stages of dehydration and exhaustion. The medical area at the Prudential Center looking like something out of the Crimean War.

God is watching the Salazars, Jose Salazar had said before the race, granting prodigious talents and expecting spectacular sac-

rifice and fidelity in return. That God has called us to great
heroism and it is within our power to accomplish it. This world
is in fact an arena for heroism, and our main task on this earth is
to be heroic.

There are those who would have us be heroic in other ways.
The marathon is foolishness. It is not truly important. It is not
rational to use it as a setting for talent and sacrifice and fidelity.
It is not the real world. Running is not our role here on earth.

Say what you will, we knew God was watching. More than
that, we ran as if God were watching. Religion is not dogma and
theology; it is not something you enunciate and systematize. It
is not even what we think we believe. It is what we do. My
religion is my truth. It is not something I have; it is something I
live. My life depends upon it.

God was watching Alberto Salazar, and he ran as if his life
depended upon it. He totally extended himself. He made the
marathon a contest between himself and the all-too-human tendency to excuse one's self and settle for less than one's best. He
pushed himself to the limit and set the example for the rest of
us. Heroism, so difficult to find in the real world, became commonplace.

God was watching Guy Gerstch, and he ran the last 19 miles
of the marathon with a fracture of his thigh bone. Guy had come
all the way from Salt Lake City and was not going to stop. That
was one reason. Deep in the subconscious was a more formidable
one. At the starting line in Hopkinton he had taken an oath. He
had given his wordless word of honor to do his absolute best. To
be a hero. He was.

God was watching Sister Madonna Buder, and she knew it.
"In the last four miles there is such a temptation to break," she
said. "I had to keep calling on Jesus to keep me running." One
hour and a half behind Alberto, this heroine finished secure in
the belief that she was pleasing the very source of creation. She
came across the line asking Divine help in this absurd human
activity.

God was watching me. His confused and wayward son. The
beauty of the marathon is that there is no indecision about what

I am supposed to do. At other times I keep asking, "Lord, what will Thou have me do?" and the answer is never clear.

In the marathon, there is no need to ask for direction. All I ask for is the strength and courage to carry it out, and the faith that it need be done. It was hours out and miles to go when I was flooded with that faith, and filled with the courage and strength to endure to the finish. I knew then a very special joy, a joy that for those moments absented me from pain. I knew myself as never before.

God was watching all of us. Consciously or subconsciously those thousands of runners felt that Presence. We are here, said the late Ernest Becker, to use ourselves up. We were meant to be heroes. We did and we were.

That is why the marathon is a serious, important and totally rational activity. It allows us to use ourselves up. To push to our limit. To be heroes. When words fail, as they so often do, it tells us what we truly believe: we have been granted prodigious talents, and spectacular sacrifices and fidelity are expected in return.

Chapter Twenty-seven
On Revealing

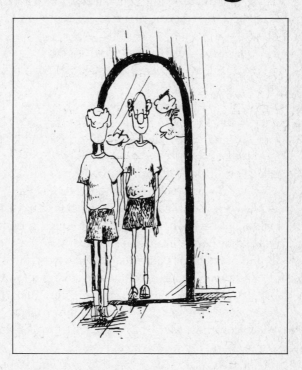

"I am a selfish person. Except, of course, for God, no one knows more about me than myself or is more interested. Whether that annoys others or not is immaterial. It is an absolute necessity. The development of the self is the first and essential step toward union with anyone else."

LATER A NATIONAL MAGAZINE described it as the world's first "Me-In." It was "The Event," which brought together speakers for the various human-potential movements for the largest self-improvement rally ever held. I was there to talk about running.

I got off to a bad start. There was a 10,000-meter race near home that I did not want to miss. So I ran the race and then arrived late for the press conference held at the luncheon break. My colleagues in this extravaganza were already explaining their positions to a skeptical crowd of reporters and writers and cameramen.

Some of the questions were frank: "What do you tell people in Queens who say this is a load of bull?" asked a New York *Daily News* reporter.

Some were snide: "If this is so important, why don't you experts do it for nothing?"

Some were far-out: "Why were the pyramids built in that shape?"

No one asked for a comment on John Leonard's column in *The New York Times*. He had no intention, wrote Leonard, of attending this gala. It was difficult enough, he said, to avoid these people at cocktail parties where they talked about nothing else but their health and their relationships. They were, he declared, graduate students in nothing more than themselves.

The press conference ended without my saying a word. The speakers went back to their chores. Drs. Masters and Johnson led off the afternoon program. I was to follow. I spent their entire session pacing nervously back and forth in the corridor behind the stage. Then my moment came.

I went out on that stage, into those bright lights, before a thousand or more people. The nervousness was gone and suddenly I was at ease. I was ready to think out loud upon the questions I never got to answer—ready to explain to myself and to the audience, to John Leonard and to the people in Queens, what running was all about.

What made it work was Buckminster Fuller. As I looked out over that expanse of faces, I saw him sitting in a separate chair placed ahead of the first row. Not 20 feet away from me, his

hands folded in his lap, his face raised expectantly, he sat .
for me to speak. This beautiful eighty-three-year-old man, whose
certainty had given me trust, sat waiting for me to say something worthwhile. And because of him, I did.

Each of us is born a genius, he had written. Each of us is born
to be a success. Somewhere things went wrong. Somewhere we
lost sight of who we were and what we could do. We became
consumed either with ambition and anxiety or boredom and
depression. We had been changed from being generalists who
knew the world into specialists who knew only a small part.

We are not to worry about the world. That was Buckminster
Fuller's message. Technology will save technology. Miniaturiza-
tion will make the world easier and easier to live in. It will be a
world that a handful of superbly intelligent people can direct.
The rest of us should concern ourselves with our own personal
salvation.

But where lay that salvation? Was there someone in this marathon of speakers able to give us that answer? Had anyone
among these authors written the ultimate how-to book? Was
there anyone whose directions we could follow to a destiny in
Paradise?

If there was, I told them, it wasn't me. I was not there, I said,
to teach them anything. I was there to make them remember
things they had forgotten. Because nothing worthwhile can be
taught. The answers to life are not in the back of the book. All
the gimmicks and techniques and the how-to books can be a
waste of time. Anything that changes your values, changes your
behavior, changes your life, has to be self-taught, must be self-
discovered. Kierkegaard was one of the first to say that. The
doleful Dane told us there is no way to communicate our deeper
experiences to another.

I agreed, I said, with the people in Queens. A lot of what
would be said today would be bull. The glow felt at this event
would be gone by tomorrow. It would last only to the extent it
moved us to action. It would be only talk unless we pushed our
bodies and minds and souls to the absolute limit. By doing and
suffering and creating, we learn—and no other way.

There is no human-potential movement worth the name if that movement does not mean growth. You have to grow to see. You have to grow to understand.

I had found that growth in running. By making running the most important thing in my life, I was able to pull my own strings, become my own best friend and realize my human potential. As I ran, I grew in health, and I grew in truth, and I grew in love.

I agreed, nevertheless, with John Leonard. I am a selfish person. Except, of course, for God, no one knows more about me than myself or is more interested. Whether that annoys others or not is immaterial. It is an absolute necessity. The development of the self is the first and essential step toward union with anyone else. To accept another, I must first accept myself. To be able to love someone else, I must first love myself.

Only rarely, however, are this acceptance and concern and love visible. I remain detached, isolated, solitary. I seek a personal perfection that shuts everyone else out. Leonard's indictment seems to stand—and behind his charge, the statement of Norman Cousins: "In our focus on individual identity and uniqueness, we have taught people to become fully involved with self, with a resultant skewing of communal values."

But once more I gazed down at Fuller's happy face and took heart. He has given us the answer. His every movement, his every word, his very presence shouts, "Life is worth living." He has the confidence that he has lived the only life cycle possible to him, has run the good race, has fought the good fight. And the young, who need no less than this faith, can see it and taste it and feel it in his very being, and love him for it.

By now the excitement had gripped me. I was brandishing the microphone, asking the audience to see this same truth. The complete realization of our self is our contribution to the common good—the greatest contribution anyone of us can make, because it is that certainty that our own life was good and true and worthwhile that gives the young what they need most: trust, the trust that they too can reach 60 and 70 and 80 with the same wonder and zest and joy.

I looked down again, and the expression on Fuller's face told me I had crossed the finish line.

A COLUMN DEFENDING the selfishness of the long-distance runner provoked an answer from my former professor of philosophy. He accepts, in part, my defense of contemplation and the solitary life. He would, up to a point, allow me to work out my salvation alone on the roads. But he insists on the additional need for devotion to the common good.

"We should not belittle one truth," he writes, "in espousing another." Contemplation is needed, he concedes, but so is the taking upon yourself the good and welfare of others. His view coincides with that of Aquinas, who stated that contemplation was one of man's highest activities. The highest, he said, was contemplation followed by implementation of the truths of that contemplation.

In fact, we are ideally suited for one or the other, not both. The religious impulse may well be resident in every man, but its manifestations are individual and even unique. This diversity is nowhere more evident than in the apparent unity of the Catholic Church. Her various religious orders run the gamut of religious expression, from the anchorite, whose mission is silence, to the missionary, whose mission is people.

Although my old teacher would take the middle ground, there is in truth very little middle ground. This is a debate that has gone on from the beginning of time.

"We should not sacrifice one good thing for another," states the professor. I agree. But he is thinking of the common good, and I am thinking of my own solitude. It is the age-old problem of being an individual and/or identifying with a group.

Join few things, wrote Frost—your family and your country and nothing between. But then Frost was also the man who said there was more religion outside the church than in.

So it goes. We are reminded of our attachment to everyone in the universe, and then we find with astonishment how much that is human is alien to us. There is always this conflict between the two points of view: the Renaissance man who says "I" and the man of the Reformation who says "We."

When I am besieged, I call upon Emerson or Thoreau or William James. "Stand apart in silence, in steadiness," counseled Emerson. "You may think I am impoverishing myself in solitude," wrote Thoreau, "but I shall burst forth a more perfect creature, fitted for a higher society."

But perhaps this struggle, and the evident truth on both sides, is most clearly seen in the relationship between James and his protégé, colleague and friend Josiah Royce.

James, in his Gifford Lectures (a series of talks given annually in Scotland by distinguished thinkers), gave his report on the religious experience. These were later to become the justly famous *Varieties of Religious Experience*—written, as he told a friend, because he believed the experience of religion was man's most important function. He also believed in man's private way to his own private truth. He was the champion of rugged individualism. This made for pluralism, the lack of absolutes. Indeed when James died, he left a note. There are no conclusions, he had written, no advice to give, no fortunes to be told.

Royce, who was as much a theologian as he was a philosopher, took exactly the opposite tack. He knew there was an Absolute, and that Absolute was God, and all this could be proven from our natural reason.

"We are saved," said Royce, "through and in the community." Our meaning, the meaning of our life, rested in loyalty—which he defined as "the willing and practical devotion of a person to a cause." Loyalty to loyalty was Royce's guiding star. It unified life, gave it center, fixity, stability.

James's loyalty was to himself, to his own truth—to his egoism versus Royce's altruism. But for all that, Royce had to be answered, and James spent the final years of his life in that intellectual effort.

"Beloved Royce," he writes at one point, "when I compose the Gifford Lecture mentally, it is with the design exclusively of overthrowing your system and ruining your peace."

He then goes on to say, "Oh, dear Royce, can I forget you or be contented out of your close neighborhood? Different as our minds are, yours has nourished mine as no other social influence has."

Royce in return called James "one of the dearest of my friends and one of the most loyal of men." And in a letter to him, he said, "No criticism of mine is hostile. Life is a sad, long road sometimes. Every friendly touch and word must be preciously guarded. I prize everything you say or do, whether I criticize or not."

This great and loving debate still goes on. There is, it seems to me, a James and Royce inside each one of us. One is at times dominant; at other times the other gains control. What we must do is reconcile these two equally positive, these two equally reproductive, drives in our lives.

The essential is that the reconciliation be a true one. It cannot be contrived. Whatever we do must be authentic. What I do must be me.

Thomas Merton once wrote to this point: "He who attempts to act and do things for others without deepening his own self-understanding, freedom, integrity and capacity to love will have nothing to give others."

Oddly, the more this push to the limits, the more the differences between us. Since I have become a runner, I see this clearly. The one thing that James and Royce shared was this demon on their backs, driving them to the best they could possibly be.

Each, of course, drove the other. "The prolonged struggle with Royce," observes scholar Ralph Barton Perry, "subjected James to a severe discipline. He had not evaded the issues. He fought them out and in doing so greatly strengthened his intellectual tissues."

And Royce was later to say, "Had I not early in my work known Professor James, I doubt whether any poor book of mine would ever be written."

So there you are. We work out our salvation in our own way, with our own truth and no one else's. The only requirement is that we be what James and Royce were—eagles.

You don't find them in flocks. Like runners, you find them one at a time.

I AM A LONER. An observer. I am one of Colin Wilson's outsiders. My involvement with other people may at times be deep and sincere, but it is nevertheless transitory. Like Thoreau, my interest and affection for my friends increases the longer I go without meeting them. Again and again, I find myself in the journals of those solitary writers over the centuries. I say the same things to myself that they confided in their notebooks.

It is nevertheless a continuing burden. I am indeed working mightily against this quality in my makeup. Every day, I roll my rock up this hill, conforming to my role in society, being a social animal. I belong to a profession whose aim is to help others. I have fathered children. I am a son and brother to others. I am a husband and part of a household. There is no end to the structures I inhabit and whose harmony depends to some extent on what I do.

Society depends upon these relationships. Tradition is the glue that holds everything in place; authority, the cement that prevents the entire structure from collapsing. There is a way things work, there is a way things are supposed to be, and there is always that second commandment of the two that can replace all others: "Love thy neighbor as thyself." So religion, too, locks me into this daily struggle between my natural tendencies and what is fitting and right and proper to do.

Even so, the self that I am cannot be denied. I see tradition as someone else's truth, not mine, and authority as an attempt to supercede my own judgment on any situation. It is something done in the interest of the community, not mine. Institutions exist because of authority. The individual must be sacrificed to the general good. And I see religion more as the exegesis—or better, the living. Religion is not something you think; it is something you do. In the end what I do may show more love of neighbor than living with them.

The Church, in prescribing celibacy for its clergy, took note of this possibility. And in its Orders, the Church acknowledges this need to be alone. There are indeed Orders whose mission is going out and preaching to all people. But there are others, like the Trappists, where life takes place in what is virtually solitary confinement.

There are deeply moral writers who speak of this ever present need to be free of others.

"I do not want to live among people who say 'we' and to be a part of 'us' to find I am at home in any human milieu, whatever it may be," writes Simone Weil. "I feel it is necessary and ordained that I should be a stranger and an exile in every human circle without exception."

"Necessary" and "ordained" are strong words. They speak of something intrinsic in the personality, the living out as fulfilling one's destiny. Nothing can stand against such a statement. There can be no argument. For Simone Weil, being a loner was being herself, the person the Creator had in mind when she was born. Our common heritage, the axioms of conduct, the accumulated scholarship of the ages, cannot withstand those forces.

You might say that Simone Weil's experience does not apply to ordinary human beings. She was certainly odd and may have been a saint. She took things much too seriously. And she had a penchant for unpopular causes—including, you might say, her own. Simone Weil, I will admit, was one of a kind, a rare bird, a museum piece.

Yet so are we all—would that each one of us could speak out for a life as distinctive as hers, that inner life that has been so suppressed and submerged we may have difficulty recognizing it, our own personal truth ready to be lived.

You may be quite surprised at the result. There are rebels yearning for tradition, revolutionaries whose need is authority. Ram Dass, after a decade of nonconformity, came back from India and announced, "The Ten Commandments is the way the world works." Your thing may be what you have been doing all your life and never fully accepted.

In all of us, there is a need for tradition and authority and religion. But each of these forces must be rooted in the self. They cannot come fully and completely from others. In all things, we must be heretics. We must, in the original Greek sense of that word, be choosers. We must choose the fitting and right true thing for us. The loner has that obligation as much as those who would bring him to the fold.

Chapter Twenty-eight
On
Believing

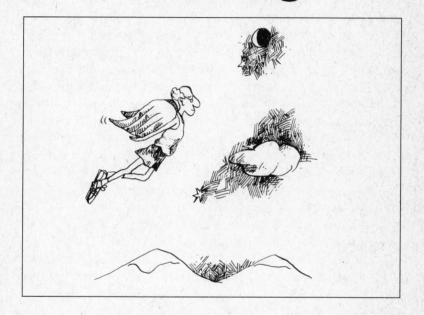

"The athlete knows he controls what happens to him. He blames no one but himself when things go wrong. The athlete makes his own luck. He decides his own fate. He believes that what he does is important and, in some odd and mystical way, matters."

"THE FREE MAN," wrote Martin Buber, "believes in destiny and that it has need of him."

More than most men, the athlete is aware of Buber's truth. The athlete knows he controls what happens to him. He blames no one but himself when things go wrong. The athlete makes his own luck. He decides his own fate. He believes that what he does is important and, in some odd and mystical way, matters.

But take us out of sport, and we see ourselves as innocent victims of forces too strong for us to handle. We are transformed from autonomous athletes to human beings completely controlled by our environment. Suddenly bureaucracy, the system, society determines what happens to us. The man who blames no one but himself in his games blames *everyone* but himself in his life.

I offer myself as Exhibit A. Take that 20-mile race in Central Park, when I won the 50-and-over plaque, beating out my perennial rival Bill Coyne at the very end of the race. I took full credit for that. And I lost my White Stag warm-up, along with my eyeglasses and car keys. For that I blamed society, the system, the Parks Department, the officials and whoever was sick enough to steal these things.

It all happened because the Parks Department's usually permissive lieutenants were replaced by some faceless commissar who would no longer let me park near the dressing room at Ninety-sixth Street. For three months I had done that, put my gear in the car and gotten a nonrunning friend to hold the keys.

This time I needed the warm-ups to jog the dozen or so blocks back up Fifth Avenue to the starting line. Now the officials got into the scenario. They offered the trunk of a car for anyone who wanted his gear brought to the finish line. Any rational man would have paused to think about the possible complications. Not I. I was on an ego trip.

Those White Stag warm-ups made me look like the runner I never was. As I jogged to the line, someone yelled, "Sheehan lives!" And then someone told me he had seen me quoted in *The New York Times Magazine* article on the Olympic marathon winner Frank Shorter.

Any playwright could have seen the tragedy unfolding: disrespect for authority, the old pride and then acting without thought of the consequences. No thinking man would let anyone but a blood relative take care of his prized warm-ups, his gold-rimmed Ben Franklin glasses and the keys to his VW. Yet in a few seconds, I reduced myself to long johns, red nylon running shorts, a ski mask and a pair of cotton gloves in a hostile city 50 miles from home.

The race was long and cruel and satisfying. Coyne went out at a pace I was afraid to match, and I never saw him again until I came upon him walking up the last hill. Running against him was like running against your best time. You knew you had to be at your best and accept pain in quantity to win. I did.

At the finish line, I changed my role from captain of my fate to victim. Our sweat suits placed with great care in the trunk had been scattered about on the grass among the crowd at the finish. Mine had disappeared. It was no wonder. Among the debris worn by my friends, the White Stag warm-up must have glittered like a Kohinoor diamond.

The end of a 20-mile race is no place to face such a crisis. The hurting after a 20-miler is sometimes worse than when you are running. This was one of those times. My legs and stomach started to cramp up as I stood there in my wet running clothes in the rapidly chilling February air.

The cramps grew worse as I got to a phone booth with a borrowed dime. They finally forced me to sit shivering on the ground, with the phone barely reaching my ear, as the family hunted for the second set of car keys 50 miles away. Two hours later I was headed home, wishing indignities on the thief and his offspring for at least three generations—and thinking of punishments for the officials and the park commissioner that Attila the Hun would have judged harsh.

Two days later I would read Buber and know that everything was my doing—or else nothing was my doing. You can't have it both ways, and I do treasure that 50-and-over plaque.

THE ATHLETE LIVES what the philosopher would explain. Epictetus said it plainly centuries ago: "If any instance of pain or pleasure, glory or disgrace be set before you, remember: now is the combat, now the Olympiad comes on, no way can it be put off, and that by one failure and defeat, honor can be lost and won."

The race is not play; it is sport. The emphasis is on the martial virtues: discipline, dedication, courage, loyalty. I am there to conquer—if not the world, myself. The race brings to the real world what is not normally in the real world: the tournament, the trial, the test by which we may come to know ourselves.

When I race, I become pure will. The race is my opportunity to suffer and to endure. In each race, I grow. I mature. And what happens in the race, I take back with me to my run. There my intellect tells me what the suffering meant. There I discover the "why" of all this doing.

The run gives me solitude for this meditation. It gives me unoccupied time—time free from people or demands or rules or regulations, time as white and virginal as new canvas, time to be used for the first and only time, time that will hold ideas as large or as small as I make them.

When I run in that time, I sometimes wonder why I race. There is no need, it seems, to go beyond this contemplation. Surely life can hold nothing better than this day-after-day communion with oneself. This is how the artist should work. This is where the writer should come upon his subject and learn how to deal with it.

True enough, I find. But sooner or later, it fails. Sooner or later, there is nothing left to write about. There are no new insights, no new experiences, no new thoughts to put on this pristine canvas. So there is a need to go back to the race, its pain and its people.

Frost said it all: "If you wish to write a poem, have an experience."

If you wish to come upon a general rule, you must first experience the particular that demonstrates that rule. If you wish to find out a quality in you or others, you must first live through an instance where that quality is demonstrated. So the race which is the microcosm of life becomes of supreme importance. If I were to run without racing I would be incomplete.

"To see complete absorption in being," writes the philosopher William Barrett, "only leads to quiescence and boring repetitions." Yet racing without running would be scurrying around, aimlessly accumulating experience without thoughts to their meaning. I would neither be growing nor learning.

Running is being, racing is doing. I have learned that truth lies in the tension between one state and the other. I know whatever stops either the running or the racing, stops the living as well.

"TO BE CONVERTED, to be regenerated, to receive grace, to experience religion," wrote William James in *The Varieties of Religious Experience*, "are so many phrases that denote the process by which a self hitherto divided and consciously wrong and inferior and unhappy, becomes unified and so consciously right and superior and happy."

James wrote at length on how and why these transformations occur, and why adolescents were particularly susceptible to this phenomenon in their behavior.

When I turned to running at forty-four, I experienced just such a conversion. For one thing, I was a forty-four-year-old adolescent. I had much the same feelings as a teenager—the same sense of incompleteness, the same sense of something missing, the same brooding, the same hope I could get through life unnoticed and therefore unpunished by my Creator.

My conversion was aided by two other motivational assets. A sense of physical sin, for one. When you are forty-four, your body becomes acutely aware of being sinned against. Another middle-aged asset is the certain knowledge that you are not doing the best that is in you, the realization that the 11th commandment is "Don't bury your talents."

When the conversion does come, it arrives in two ways. The first is preoccupation with sin. This is conversion due to guilt—my guilt about what I had done to the person I had been. This conversion is conscious and voluntary. It is quite clear what must be done, and I must simply summon the willpower to do it.

In such instances, James wrote, the regenerative change is usually gradual and consists in building the new "I" piece by piece. That "I" is the person I was before I became the person who began running—an "I" that I could no longer accept. I could see my sins and was ready to repent.

There are fitness evangelists who preach physical sin. They have their own ten commandments of do's and don'ts. When they face a smoking, drinking, overweight, out-of-shape audience, you are reminded of Cotton Mather working over his New England congregation. Such revival meetings frequently harvest a bushel of souls ready to run and sin no more.

I go through that conversion every time I am out on the roads. When the sweating starts, I can feel the badness leaving me. I can sense the excess fat being burned off, the training effect on the heart. I am aware of the strength and endurance building in my muscles. I am purging myself of sin, ridding myself of guilt.

There is, however, another and more subtle conversion going on—a conversion that ultimately produces what James called "the state of assurance" and Maslow defined as "the peak experience." By any name, it is the happening that convinces us we are indeed whole and happy and one with the universe.

This conversion is not a movement away from sin. It is a movement toward righteousness, toward the positive ideal we wish to attain, toward the splendor each one of us was created to attain. This is a conversion that is going on in the subconscious, in our subliminal life. It is therefore involuntary. It is accomplished not by willpower, but by relaxation and acceptance and self-surrender.

In this conversion, the impetus is not guilt but shame—shame that I have not taken out of every moment what was there to be done, shame that I have fallen short of my own potential.

Yet this type of conversion is a positive one. I become excited not about my faults, but my excellence, not about what I have done but what I can do, not about who I was but who I will be.

All this requires, said James, an active interior life. I have found that in running. Somewhere in the second half-hour, especially with the wind at my back, I can enter my cell and meditate. Motion has become my mantra, and my subconscious is in ferment. Not that all or most of it surfaces or is plainly seen, but on the infrequent occasions that it does surface I realize what has been percolating in those recesses.

I am out on the roads several days a week renewing my vows, hoping for those signs given the elect.

My conversion is a series of conversions. I must continue with my fight with physical sin; I must trust that my subconscious will continue its path toward my perfection and on occasion permit me a glimpse or two.

James summarized this well. First, that state of assurance. The main characteristic, he said, is the loss of all worry—the sense that all is ultimately well, the peace, the harmony, the willingness-to-be.

Converts, James said, have a sense of perceiving things not known before. The world seems different now. There is a feeling as if everything is being seen for the first time. And finally, there is that ecstasy of happiness produced.

Why, I sometimes ask myself, must all this occur only on the roads? What is it that makes running an essential of this whole phenomenon? Is it the solitude or the motion or both that are the source of this revelation?

Whatever the reason, Emerson was familiar with this sort of occurrence. In *The Transcendentalist* he wrote, "[My faith] is a certain brief experience, which surprised me on the highway and made me aware that I had played the fool among fools—that I should never be fool more. Yet in the space of an hour, I was at my old tricks—a selfish member of a selfish society."

So each time I run, it is to become, if only briefly, the person the Lord meant me to be—unified and consciously right and superior and happy.

Epilogue
Beyond
Fitness

"Fitness helps you look for the life you should
lead. Being an athlete means you have
found it."

BEING FIT IS ONE THING. Being an athlete is another. Thirty
minutes of movement done at a comfortable pace four times a
week will make you fit. The movement could be running, cycling,
swimming or walking. Two hours a week will make you fit. But
athletes who are runners, cyclists, swimmers or walkers may
train those two hours *every day*.

Fitness is the ability to do work. There is a relationship between the time put in and the energy derived from it. Fitness is
a scientific, measurable, testable fact. People who want it can be
told just how much it will cost. Time and again, researchers have
proven the validity of the fitness equation of duration, intensity
and frequency.

Being an athlete is something quite different. Fitness is what
you pass through on the way to a superior physical and mental
and spiritual state. Beyond fitness is also a new and demanding,
albeit infinitely rewarding, life-style.

Fitness is keeping the commandments. Being an athlete is
pushing one's physical capabilities to the limit, getting the most

out of one's genetic endowment. Fitness is attention to the minimum daily requirements of the body. Being an athlete is attaining the maximum daily output—and paying what it costs.

Fitness and its maintenance can be programmed. You can allot a half-hour of your daily schedule for the necessary activity. Some run in the morning so they can then concentrate on their work the rest of the day. Most find a time that interferes the least with other more interesting and important activities.

The athlete, on the other hand, looks for a time when other less interesting and important activities interfere least with his or her sport. Play, not work, has the priority.

Being an athlete is not something I do an hour or so a day. It is something I *am*. Being a runner is something that informs my entire day. My 24 hours is lived as a runner. Everything that occurs takes on increased interest and importance in so much as it pertains to my running. My entire environment, internal and external, is monitored in relation to effect on my performance. So I am now runner-doctor, runner-writer, runner-lecturer. I am runner-father, runner-husband, runner-friend. For me, fitness is no longer enough. I must be an athlete.

Fitness helps you look for the life you should lead. Being an athlete means you have found it.